To
Wrestle
With Demons

A Psychiatrist Struggles
to Understand
His Patients and Himself

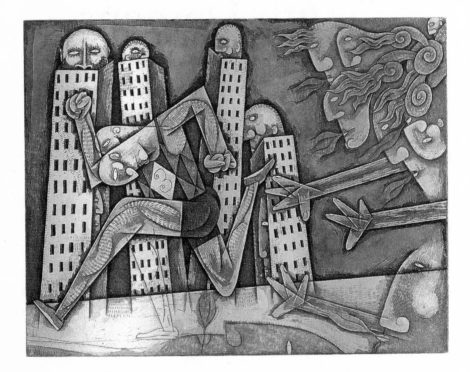

To
Wrestle
With Demons

*A Psychiatrist Struggles
to Understand
His Patients and Himself*

By

Keith Russell Ablow, M.D.

Foreword by
Robert Coles

Illustrations by
Richard Downs

American
Psychiatric
Press, Inc.

Washington, DC
London, England

Note: The author has worked to ensure that all information in this book concerning drug dosages, schedules, and routes of administration is accurate as of the time of publication and consistent with standards set by the U.S. Food and Drug Administration and the general medical community. As medical research and practice advance, however, therapeutic standards may change. For this reason and because human and mechanical errors sometimes occur, we recommend that readers follow the advice of a physician who is directly involved in their care or the care of a member of their family.

Some circumstantial details of case histories have been changed to ensure confidentiality.

Copyright © 1992 Keith Russell Ablow, M.D.
ALL RIGHTS RESERVED
Manufactured in the United States of America on acid-free paper.
First Edition
95 94 93 92   4 3 2 1

American Psychiatric Press, Inc.
1400 K Street, N.W., Washington, DC 20005

Library of Congress Cataloging-in-Publication Data
Ablow, Keith R.
     To wrestle with demons :   a psychiatrist struggles to understand
his patients and himself /   by Keith Russell Ablow.
         p.   cm.
     ISBN 0-88048-546-9
     1. Psychiatry—Philosophy.   2. Ablow, Keith R.—Philosophy.
3. Ablow, Keith R.—Anecdotes.   4. Psychiatrists—Anecdotes.
I. Title.
     [DNLM: 1. Psychiatry—personal narratives.   WZ 112.5.P6 A152t]
     RC437.5.A24 1992
     616.89′001—dc20
DNLM/DLC   92-10468
for Library of Congress   CIP

British Library Cataloguing in Publication Data
A CIP record is available from the British Library.

No one who, like me, conjures up the most evil
of those half-tamed demons that inhabit the
human breast, and seeks to wrestle with them,
can expect to come through the struggle
unscathed.

Sigmund Freud

This book is dedicated to Drs. Carol Nadelson, Theodore Nadelson, and Henry Seidel. In making a physician of me, they wasted not a splinter of whatever timber I could bring them.

Contents

Acknowledgments   *xi*

Foreword   *xiii*
   Robert Coles

Preface   *xv*

Mazes of the Mind

1	Exploring Mazes of the Mind	3
2	When Dancing Naked Feels Like Home	9
3	Life Stories	15
4	Acting Out	21
5	Electroshock	27
6	What Kind of Cure?	33
7	Ranging Far From Reality	39

An Examined Life

8	Reaping the Benefits of an Examined Life	47
9	Personal Connections	53
10	Ambivalence	59
11	The Last Night On Call	65
12	Saying Goodbye With Grace	71

Gates

13 The Gatekeeper   79

14 Sex in Psychotherapy   85

15 One of the Boys   91

16 Fatal Afflictions   97

17 Souled: Money and Therapy   103

18 Ministering to the Spirit   109

My Brother's Keeper

19 My Brother's Keeper: The Dilemmas of
    Medical Guardianship   117

20 The Mask of Mania   123

21 Danger   129

22 Murder With No Apparent Motive   135

23 Mental State   141

24 Moral Insanity: Character and Mental Illness   147

25 Safe Passage: Psychotherapy and the Status Quo   153

Acknowledgments

All but one of the essays in this book have appeared in *The Washington Post*. Sandra G. Boodman and Abigail Trafford, my artist-editors there, have earned my appreciation and trust, and my friendship.

I am deeply grateful to Robert Coles for providing his foreword. Having my writing introduced so warmly by a man whose work has been an inspiration to me is a precious reward.

My thanks also to Carol Nadelson, M.D., Ronald E. McMillen, Claire Reinburg, Julie Glass, Pam Harley, Jane Hoover Davenport, Greg Kuny, Karen Loper and Cary Wyman of the American Psychiatric Press, Inc. What a rare comfort it has been to put my words in their good hands.

Finally, I thank my family. It was, no doubt, their love that first convinced me of the power of that which cannot be seen.

Foreword

I worry sometimes about the future of psychoanalysis," I heard Anna Freud remark toward the end of her life—and then I braced myself for an elderly woman's recitation of all the ills to which a younger generation is heir. But she had a surprise in store for those of us ready to lament her inability to avoid a certain kind of egoistic sentimentality. Instead of issuing a lamentation for the wonderful days of yore, now receding even from the memories of fast-diminishing survivors, she spoke of her hope for the future, a hope she connected, interestingly enough, to individuals, rather than theoretical breakthroughs, new strategies or methodologies: "It is true, psychoanalysis no longer commands the attention it used to—and frankly, I think that is a good thing. We can do our work without having people breathing down our necks! I am often asked, these days, what I see ahead for our work, and I say, always: a bright future—it rests on the younger people who are attracted to our field. I think of certain ones [of these 'younger' people], and I am grateful to them, very glad they are here."

I thought of that poignant moment repeatedly as I read Keith Ablow's wonderfully lucid, touching and edifying collection of essays— in their sum, a young psychiatrist's affirmation of a calling, a vocation. He is, I think, the kind of psychiatrist Miss Freud at her best would have enjoyed getting to know—independent-minded, broadly educated, thoughtful and compassionate: the kind of psychiatrist, to go further, a patient would want to get to know. By no means, unfortunately, does one make that statement about every psychiatrist, even those well trained and duly accredited. In every profession there are those young ones who obey and comply, until they graduate or fulfill their requirements, and then take their marching orders from various "principalities and powers." Psychiatry, too, can become an instrument of such conformity and compliance—even as it can lend itself to the larger world as a normative agent of sorts: shape up, behave like "us," or get called "sick," "deviant" and "abnormal." For Dr. Ablow, as he makes clear again and again, the dangers of such a way of thinking (or *being*, actually) are substantial indeed: the doctor becomes the ultimate victim—robbed of his or her freedom to think critically, to be his or her own judge as to what a particular patient needs, how that patient ought be regarded.

These essays tell us much about the continuing struggles of one doctor to learn about himself—what it is in him that heals, what it is in him that can become an obstacle to healing. As one goes through the essays, one gets to know both an individual and a contemporary profession—the privileges and opportunities, the hazards and temptations that can all too readily set the stage for clinical successes or failures. One also gets to know a lot about the rest of us who live in late-20th-century secular America—we who so often turn to psychiatrists not only out of our personal difficulties or problems, but in search of some sense of life's meaning and purpose. As Dr. Ablow reminds us, psychological and psychiatric territory adjoins the moral and spiritual turf to which other professions lay claim.

Most of all, these essays, in a quiet and unassuming manner, attest to the growing wisdom achieved by a doctor who started out with all sorts of ideas, preconceptions, ambitions, assumptions, and quite simply (but it is, really, not simple at all, of course) let himself become not only the knowing and able physician, but once again, the student who has ever so much to learn. The teachers, needless to say, were not only the supervisors or fellow residents whom we meet in the pages that follow, but very important, one patient after another, men and women whose trials and tribulations become, after a fashion, their psychiatrist's, and who, unbeknownst to themselves, perhaps, became his very good and patient teachers. The result is a young psychiatrist of ideals, of good values; a psychiatrist unfettered by various orthodoxies, able to think for himself, even as he is respectful of what others, near and far in space and time, have (or have had) to offer; a psychiatrist who hasn't lost his common sense, who doesn't feel compelled to embrace every passing fad, and who (a welcome virtue for his readers) knows how to think clearly and set down lucid, vigorous prose, uncluttered by pretentious, murky jargon. Altogether, a welcome event, indeed: Keith Ablow's book as a reminder to us that a profession not without its detractors (or its all too eager and zealous partisan defenders—maybe two sides of the same coin) can still offer us the kind of wise, reflective mind patients will continue to need over the years.

Robert Coles
Harvard University
Cambridge, Massachusetts

Preface

If I have seen further . . . it is by standing on the shoulders of
Giants.

Sir Isaac Newton

One core question has informed my work on each of the essays in
this collection: *How can I share the gifts that psychiatry has given me?*
This question not only has guided me nightly to my writing desk,
sometimes embracing me until morning, but has given me direction and
courage at those moments when the fear of self-disclosure—a pestilence
as destructive as any other—has threatened to choke off my voice,
leaving you and me strangers.

My expectations as I began psychiatry training were not meager. I
wanted to become facile in the art of diagnosis and the use of medications. I felt the need to be present and helpful at moments of uncertainty
and pain in the lives of others. And I had hope that the field might read
me a kind of running drama of human stories.

All this has happened. I have soaked up the signs and symptoms of
the approximately 300 psychiatric disorders constantly being defined
and redefined in our evolving diagnostic manual. I have looked through
windows on the brain opened by research and technology and can almost
visualize the brain's chemical messengers, their target receptors and the
medications that sculpt them. I know many of the intricacies of match-
ing highly effective pharmacologic cures to the illnesses that afflict my
patients. I have had hundreds of individuals look to me for comfort and
expertise as gripping chapters in their lives unfolded.

I have had quiet time to reflect on psychiatry's development as a
field, with roots in morality and ethics and towering branches into the
neurosciences. I have wondered over its intricate applications in settings
as varied as public and private psychiatric wards, medical and surgical
wards, outpatient clinics, emergency rooms and courtrooms.

But so much more has happened—and here, the unexpected part—
to *me*. I can hear and feel the music between spoken words, a silent and

explosive score, where I once would have sworn there was none. I have been witness to irresistible proofs that the unconscious is at work in each of us, making the earliest pages of our life stories animate in those we pen today and will pen tomorrow. I know now that we are connected, one to another, in complex, perhaps inexplicable, ways we know precious little about. I believe deeply that empathy, properly harnessed, can heal. I have found wonder at the interface of the brain and the mind.

These insights have been gifts from my patients, colleagues and supervisors. They are my Giants. There have been glistening threads—a young immigrant who admitted to missing the voices my medicines took away, a grandmother whose feet burned relentlessly for her grandson fighting in a distant desert, a teacher of mine brought to tears describing what he loved in his work. There have also been terribly dark threads—a patient's suicide, violence against me, the murder of my friend and fellow resident in psychiatry. The fabric of what I thought would be a profession, plain and simple, has blanketed my whole being. I am a different person than I was just four years ago.

The pages that follow are my best attempt to share the knowledge that has changed me. Not infrequently I spent 30 or more hours on a single essay, challenging myself to surrender thoughts that initially pleaded to stay inside me, making the seductive case that they should remain part of the profession's private trust. I give them to you so that you might be warmed, as I have been, by the certain knowledge that we are more alike than different in our needs and fears and much more alone than we need to be.

Keith Russell Ablow, M.D.
Chelsea, Massachusetts

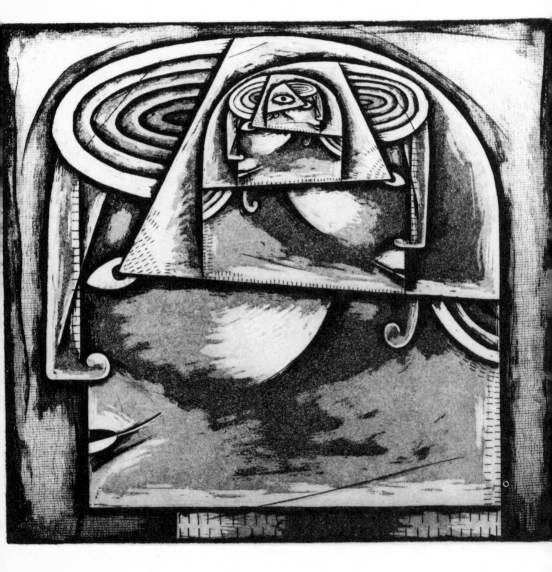

Mazes of the Mind

1

Exploring
Mazes
of the Mind

Inside every patient, there's a poet trying to get out.

Anatole Broyard   "Doctor Talk to Me"
New York Times Magazine 1990

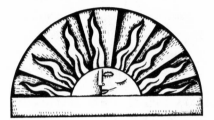

Treating psychiatric patients is hard to talk about, in the way that the soul is hard to talk about. There is something immeasurable in the work, a coalescence of mind and spirit, that resists words. I think the resistance to discuss the psychiatrist's trade is due not so much to its complexity as it is to the practitioner's fear—my fear—that the beauty in it will evaporate if we examine it too closely; as if, by explaining the workings of empathy, we will explain it away. Maybe that's the reason for all the infighting between those who understand mental illnesses in terms of disordered life stories and others who understand them as abnormal brain chemistry.

I used to be more comfortable with the chemistry myself. As a medical student at Johns Hopkins, the scientist in me readily accepted the notion that hallucinations sprang from too much of a neurotransmitter called dopamine and that depression was a disorder of two more called norepinephrine and serotonin. I pictured antipsychotic drugs blocking chemical receptors in the brain and antidepressants flooding them. The success of electroconvulsive therapy reassured me that mental illness was a kind of faulty chemical wiring between neurons. It made me feel vulnerable to these illnesses because accidents of biology could happen to anyone.

All of that, of course, is true. Most mental illnesses do have something to do with disordered chemicals in the brain, and faulty wiring like that can happen to anyone. Many patients do, thankfully, get better on the right combination of medicines. But as it turns out, that is not the whole story. It may not be half the story. And only recently have I learned to listen closely enough to my patients, residents of a spartan, locked ward at a Boston state hospital, for them to tell me the rest.

The rest is about what happens to people when their needs for affection and security and understanding are unmet. It is about desperate survival strategies patients use to provide some insulation against the chaos of their lives.

I learned part of this by listening to a patient, a recent immigrant in his twenties. He was committed because he heard voices that told him to do everything from setting fire to his bed to overdosing on aspirin— both of which he had done. He told me he felt sad and that he couldn't sleep and had no appetite.

Everything fit well with what's called depression with psychotic features, an illness of mood that can include either hallucinations or bizarre and unshakable beliefs. People with the disorder not only feel sad but also can see visions or hear voices. They can come to believe they are responsible for all the evil in the world. I spent a long time picking out an antipsychotic and an antidepressant medication that I thought might work. And in a couple of weeks, the voices were gone. The patient said he felt better. I agreed he was ready to go home.

The problem was that as soon as he left the hospital, he stopped taking those medicines. Psychiatrists call that noncompliance, and the word was all over the paperwork from the emergency room he ended up in, having overdosed, again, on aspirin. The doctors made sure he was medically stable, then sent him back to my ward.

"If you don't take your pills," I explained, "the voices will come back."

"I know," he said quietly. "No voices with medicine."

"So, we'll start the medicine, again."

He looked down. "I want to keep them," he whispered.

"Keep what?"

"The voices." He noticed my surprise and smiled. "Just the good ones."

The good voices, it turns out, generally talked to each other, not to my patient. Sometimes, he couldn't even make out what they were saying. But they still made him feel less alone in his tiny rented room, a room as far from the American dream he'd heard about as it was from his homeland. My treatment had taken those voices away, along with

6

the "bad voices" that told him to hurt himself, and he couldn't live so utterly alone.

I might not be able to, either. That's where the sadness I felt at the time must have been coming from. And that sadness was as important a therapeutic tool as the medicine. It allowed me to see how his life story had shaped his illness and complicated its treatment. He wasn't just sick; he was sick and defeated and alone. The three things had become one; he needed help with all of them.

That doesn't sound very scientific. I was so prepared to embrace the medical model that I doubted these connections even as I recognized them. But they happen and, like it or not, their utility resists biomedical interpretation. The art of psychiatry is in marrying empathy and science in service to the patient.

I learned more about this from another patient, a 30-year-old woman with schizophrenia. She was admitted after assaulting a relative. For the first week of her hospitalization, our longest meeting lasted four minutes. That was how long it took me to begin explaining again how her drug abuse was worsening her hallucinations and making her violent. As if on cue, she would stand up, announce that she wasn't ill at all and walk out of my office.

I called several of the other hospitals where she had been treated. No one knew much about her other than which medicines she'd been given. No one had been able to sit with her long enough. But buried in 10-year-old records from her first hospitalization was one short paragraph about her evolving talent as an artist.

Our next meeting wasn't about illness at all; it was about painters she admired. It lasted half an hour. Two meetings later, we were talking about the steady hand needed for portraiture and how her medicine made her shake.

"Your illness has taken a lot from you," I said. Most antipsychotic drugs do have physical side effects, some of which can't be easily managed.

"It's taken my whole life away, really," she answered. "The drugs just help me forget."

Try to listen to the schizophrenic drug user without listening to the painter, and you might as well be in the room alone.

After enough lessons from patients like these, I've started developing what some people call a third ear. I have begun to listen not only to the patient but to myself listening to the patient, feeling connections as an omniscient observer might. I stop frequently and think, "Why is it that I feel angry sitting with this patient?" Or anxious? Or happy?

I ask the patient questions designed to fill in my own emotional blanks. And the beautiful thing is that in doing so, I've ended up learning about both of us.

2

When Dancing Naked
Feels Like Home

I says, "Maybe it ain't a sin. Maybe it's just the way folks is.
Maybe we been whippin' the hell out of ourselves for
nothin'." An' I thought how some sisters took to beatin'
theirselves with a three-foot shag of bobwire. An' I thought
how maybe they liked to hurt themselves, an' maybe I liked
to hurt myself. Well, I was layin' under a tree when I figured
that out, and I went to sleep. And it come night an' it was
dark when I come to. They was a coyote squawkin' near by.
Before I knowed it, I was sayin' out loud, "The hell with it!
There ain't no sin and there ain't no virtue. There's just stuff
people do. It's all part of the same thing. And some of the
things folks do is nice, and some ain't nice, but that's as far
as any man got a right to say."

John Steinbeck   *The Grapes of Wrath*

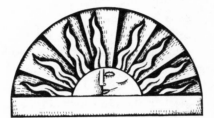

I did not begin training as a psychiatrist with an open mind.

As strange as it might seem for someone beginning a career based on insight, I had resolved not to change. I was frightened that my personality might be pasteurized by the process, that forces would make of me a blank slate on which others would feel free to write their life stories.

Worse yet, I feared becoming eccentric—even driven crazy—by listening to troubled or mentally ill people. It is testimony to the tenacity of the caricature of the field that this fear survived my close and valued relationships with my mentors in medical school, psychiatrists who were not just personable, but charismatic.

I resolved to keep a vigil of sorts. My interests then ran much closer to pharmacology than to Freud, so I thought it would be easy to skate safely over the contrived meanings that others might coax me to find in everyday speech or events. I would be particularly alert for uninvited analysis of my personal style. I would emerge untouched.

But for all my plans and the energy I expended to keep my distance, I have been swept up by my work. My patients and supervisors have helped me to hear and to feel an undercurrent of meaning in human interactions that is as subtle as it is powerful.

Recently an elderly patient of mine arrived for her appointment, then sat down and insisted it would be her last visit. She said that terminating therapy before we had planned should not matter to me, as ours was a business-like relationship. "You can't care too much about your patients," she asserted, "or you won't have a life."

"You're worried you'll keep me from having my own life?" I asked. "Isn't that what you said last week about your son?"

"You remind me of him," she said.

"And he moved away."

"Well, how long are you planning to stick around?" she asked.

A year ago, I would have heard a simple goodbye in a mother's sadness at not seeing her son. But these connections have occurred with such frequency and emotional force that I can no longer deny them. The harmony or dissonance that plays in the background of a conversation is becoming as loud as the words.

When a valued colleague overslept and missed a recent presentation of mine, I wondered whether we had become too competitive. A friend spent more money than he should on a sculpture, and I warned him that debt could be his way of avoiding change, binding himself to his lucrative, but unfulfilling, job—just like his father.

The unstated messages and intentions in actions and words sometimes seem so obvious to me that I feel embarrassed for the person communicating them, as though I am eavesdropping on a private struggle between the conscious and unconscious.

I often agonize about whether I should share my interpretations when they arise in social situations with people outside the office. Often, I do not. I don't want to impose my uninvited introspection on others, knowing that it can bring great pain and tremendous anger. That's why people have defenses against their emotions.

I had imagined that after listening to my patients' problems, I would shrink from wanting to hear about those of my friends or acquaintances. I would have given all my empathy at the office, and would welcome shooting the breeze.

But the opposite has happened. I am uncomfortable on the surface of a discussion, saddened when a conversation is limited to pleasantries. My training and experience have taught me that everyone is in some sort of pain, and that whenever I expend the time and energy to look, I find it. Whether the problem is a strained relationship, an unrealized goal, a denied passion or a fear of death, everything is not all right.

I am less and less able to walk away from the tug of doubt I feel when the answers to my questions, whether put to a patient or a friend, seem convenient or simplistic.

At a restaurant several weeks ago a group of friends and I were joined by a woman we had recently met. I asked how her day had been. "Like the rest of them," she smiled. "I need a beer."

The group chuckled, then quickly went back to arguing about the World Series.

Most of me went along. "Well, how are the rest of them?" I wanted to ask.

I didn't, because I am not willing to pay the price, which I imagine might include social ostracism, the reputation of being the chink in everyone's emotional armor.

Listening to people's pain has connected me to the suffering of others. I understand that what looks like free choice in an adult can have its roots in childhood trauma. A woman who repeatedly engages in abusive relationships, for example, may be replaying a childhood tragedy of abuse at her father's hand, trying to understand it or, perhaps, to finally achieve a measure of control over it.

Recently I went to a bachelor party for an old friend and ended up talking to the topless dancer. "You like this job?" I asked.

"I love it," she said. "The first time I stepped onto the runway, I felt so at home."

I couldn't resist. "What was home like?" I asked.

I have been told that what is happening to me is just a self-indulgent version of weakness. An older friend of mine, greatly skilled at leveraged buyouts, warned me I am losing my competitive edge. He has a gambler's eye for opportunity. "You have to understand," he explained, "that some people come to the table to lose. That's the reason they are there."

There's an element of truth in what he says. Some people who feel worthless, who have learned in one way or another that the world is cruel or capricious, will go about proving it to themselves, again and again. But I cannot abide it at my table. I have chosen the role of helping people make the most of their cards, even when they seem hellbent on folding.

I have become convinced that most unhealthy patterns are never interrupted, that pain is commonly buried, that terrible guilt routinely lies unacknowledged to fester. What my patients tell me, I imagine my colleagues' patients tell them. I hear hints of some of the same unresolved issues in my friends, and I recognize them in myself. The code of silence around all this frustrates me because the truth is that, although we won't tell each other, we are more alike than different in our needs and fears. We are much more alone than we need to be.

About halfway through my inpatient work at a Boston state psychiatric hospital, I went searching for a passage in Steinbeck's *Grapes of Wrath*. The gist of it had stuck with me from years earlier. The words are those of a preacher who has left the cloth:

"The hell with it! There ain't no sin and there ain't no virtue. There's just stuff people do. It's all part of the same thing. And some of the things folks do is nice, and some ain't nice, but that's as far as any man got a right to say."

Touching the pain I work with feels very much like love. The fact that I have had the opportunity to sit with a homeless schizophrenic man or a pregnant intravenous drug user and find their fears—of failure and loneliness and death and, yes, insanity—in myself has brought me to tears. As different as our lives are, we know something about one another. In listening to suffering that others had warned would drag me down, I have been lifted to a new optimism, a conviction that human beings are connected by a core goodness that may lie just below the surface.

This goodness, interestingly enough, is not revealed to me in success. I feel there is nothing so honest or beautiful as the connections I have been privileged to make with those who are utterly lost.

3

Life Stories

What sort of future is coming up from behind I don't really know. But the past, spread out ahead, dominates everything in sight.

Robert M. Pirsig
Zen and the Art of
Motorcycle Maintenance

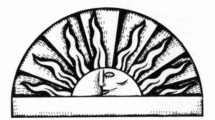

The idea that a person's past could unconsciously and dramatically influence the present used to make me smirk.

As a medical student, delving deep into a patient's early experiences was the part of psychiatry that seemed the most eccentric and the least doctorly. I suspected that the whole notion of unconscious connections between past and present was a powerful myth spun by creative minds who had broken with scientific process and wandered to guesswork. I, on the other hand, would keep my feet firmly grounded in fact.

But listening to my patients has proven me wrong. Again and again, decisions they make turn out to have undeniable connections with earlier experiences in their lives. It is as if forgotten or seemingly disconnected chapters in their life stories continue to influence the evolving plots.

One patient came to the clinic seeking treatment for extreme stress. His second marriage was to a chronically sick woman whose care took almost all his time. "I'm at the end of my rope," he said. "I'm wearing myself out running to doctors, making sure she takes her medicines, taking the kids out so she can rest. I'm beat." He had been married previously to a woman who ultimately died from a disease that was already taking its toll when they met.

During our fourth meeting, my patient's devotion to these ill women began to take the tone of servitude. He described the responsibility as inescapable—as if he was destined to forever be both husband and nurse.

"Did anyone get sick in your family when you were a child? Or die?" I asked.

"No, no one. Why?" he asked.

"Anyone?" I pressed. "A friend, maybe?"

"Well, sure. Now that you mention it. My best friend in fourth grade . . . ," he said, then fell silent for a few moments, his eyes welling with tears. "We were like the same person, see? I remember going to visit him in the hospital."

"What was that like for you?" I asked.

"The worst thing wasn't all the tubing they'd stuck in him," he said. "It was this nurse who kept telling me, 'There's nothing you can do. There's nothing you can do.'"

The plot made irresistible sense. Having been told as a boy that he could do nothing to save such a precious friend, my patient seemed to be desperately engaging illness in battle as a man.

Part of the evidence that an unconscious link with the past is truly at the heart of a current behavior pattern is the patient's response when the connection is uncovered. There is often a moment of astonishment or embarrassment that the relationship could have gone unnoticed so long, the sudden flash of recognition similar to the response of encountering an old friend while traveling in a distant land—a *"What are you doing here?"* look.

A woman who was ending a friendship of 20 years described the relationship as "one-sided." She said she had suffered through decades of supporting her friend emotionally, without the effort being reciprocated.

"Why have you decided to end the friendship now, after so long?" I asked.

"The final straw," she said, "was when she told me I'd have to cancel my trip to see her because her son would be visiting unexpectedly. There's only one spare bedroom. I said I'd be happy to sleep on the couch, but she wouldn't hear of it."

It turned out that the woman had grown up in a family in which she and her siblings had to be adopted. Although she begged to be placed with her sister, none of the adoptive families had room for two children.

When she related the memory of her sadness to me, she suddenly grasped her forehead. She seemed surprised. "When my friend didn't have room for me to visit, it was just like that, wasn't it? That's why it hurt so much."

Seemingly independent experiences can even cause destructive patterns that include physical symptoms. Months ago, I treated a man who endured bouts of fear, heart palpitations and sweating whenever his relationship with a woman seemed on the brink of marriage. His heart proved to be perfectly healthy. But three times, his condition became severe enough that the women he loved abandoned him.

In talking about his childhood, he told me of his mother's cruelty. "She'd say, 'Come here, my sweetheart,' and, then, when I did, she'd slap me across the face." That vivid image from the past seemed like part of the explanation for the patient's recurrent symptoms. It made sense that being repeatedly seduced and violently rejected by his mother could make him panic at the thought of confessing love. It could also lead him to test the affection of a mate by requiring a demonstration of unwavering commitment—like sticking by him through worsening illness.

Insight-oriented psychotherapy presumes the existence of a core self with real hopes, needs and emotions that can be misdirected or thwarted by invisible anchors to past traumas, as though the mind is stuck in an oscillating circuit, repeating destructive patterns endlessly.

By connecting forgotten or seemingly unrelated experiences with present emotions and decisions, psychiatrists hope that patients will be free to chart a truer course.

The first man I described, for example, might allow himself more freedom from his current role as his wife's caretaker. He might better understand his motivation should there come a time when he considers commitment to another debilitated woman.

The woman who decided to end her friendship might reevaluate how much of her anger can be traced to her earlier abandonment. She might wonder whether she seeks out relationships in which she is consistently the more giving partner. And, rather than breaking off, she might be able to help her friend understand her true need for support and reassurance.

Sometimes, people feel that the easy way out is to forget pain, to let "sleeping dogs lie." But keeping the past buried is not a passive process. It takes mental energy to suppress the painful memories that lead to unhealthy patterns.

One patient, locked in repeated, exhausting struggles with authority figures, had been recounting her physical abuse as a child. When we began touching on the most hurtful aspects, she became evasive. Eventually, she took to starting each therapy session with a long rendition of how her day had been spent. Sometimes, she wandered into her opinion of world events.

"You seem to be spending a lot of your energy and our time avoiding the painful topic we've been talking about," I finally commented.

"I keep running into corners, and you keep trying to flush me out," she said.

Exactly. By exposing memories that wreak havoc under cover, the energy of running away—whether to one's daily routine or to unhealthy relationships—can be better directed.

As a psychiatrist, I must remain cautious as I settle on these understandings of how earlier chapters in my patients' lives are influencing their present emotions or behaviors. If the connections I identify make no sense to them, they will have little value to the people I am trying to help.

I may press my point by reviewing the evidence for the connection or introducing consistent new evidence as it unfolds. But other times I come to feel, far from my patient being resistant, the scenario I have presented has no inherent power to move him or her. The only thing separating fiction from truth in a patient's life story is, in fact, that individual's sense of whether the plot *feels* right, not whether it is historically accurate.

Knowing precisely when to abandon my version of a patient's life story is difficult because there is no way to objectively confirm or refute it. The original manuscript is unavailable. I can never know for sure whether a patient's protest against a connection I propose represents a well-defended fortress or is simple honesty. Furthermore, my own life story will influence which themes I identify as compelling, those which I am happy to skim over and those which never occur to me at all.

I look for hints in my patient's behavior. Tears, surprise or anger at a connection I propose makes me want to delve deeper. So, too, does a knee-jerk or impassioned rejection. If the patient misses the next appointment, I wonder whether I have hit a raw and true nerve or whether I have wandered hopelessly afar. Considered skepticism makes me feel most strongly that I am off base.

The truth in psychotherapy is ultimately what *feels* true. The facts are subjective. That doesn't bother me anymore. The validity of the connections I uncover is determined by whether they alleviate my patients' pain and improve their lives.

4

Acting Out

The human understanding is like a false mirror, which, receiving rays irregularly, distorts and discolors the nature of things by mingling its own nature with it.

Francis Bacon *Novum Organum*

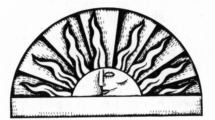

*B*eginning treatment with a psychiatric patient feels like walking onstage in a play, never having read the script and waiting for hints about the role. No wonder my inclination is to keep quiet and listen.

Psychiatrists sometimes describe the use of silence as "letting it happen." Much of the *it* is a phenomenon known as transference: The patient unconsciously develops irrational feelings toward the therapist that actually stem from other relationships, often early in life.

One of my patients was a woman who had telephoned the clinic director seeking treatment for an episode of severe depression. We had never seen each other, nor even spoken by phone. She followed me from the waiting area, took a seat in my office and tried to smile through gathering tears. I looked at her questioningly.

"The minute I saw you out there with the other doctors," she explained, "I told my friend, 'I hope I don't get that one. He's a low-life.'"

It turned out that the patient had been abused and then abandoned by her father when she was young. She had replayed that trauma through a series of romances with abusive men. And she had already grafted that experience onto our relationship.

Many weeks later, faced with an emergency, I canceled one of our meetings. She reacted angrily.

"You blew me off!" she said later. She tried to retreat from the anger immediately. "You'd really be in trouble if I knew where you lived," she laughed.

"Are you really angry enough to hurt me?" I asked.

"Don't be such a psychiatrist," she taunted. "You're hardly the first guy to stand me up."

"Who was the first?"

She considered the question briefly. "I guess my father."

It is not surprising that a woman trying to contain nearly overwhelming rage at her father might run from it—to dependency or depression or even suicide—rather than acting on it. The mind then buries the connection deeper and deeper, even as seepage from that forgotten ground contaminates everything around it.

Part of my job is to serve as a lightning rod for these unresolved emotional issues. If I can inspire trust, my patients may be able to play out their unconscious conflicts with me, slowly understanding and making peace with them.

Pacing is important. Transference can be powerful to the point of being uncontrollable. A gay man I treated early in my training expressed a desire to leave his long-term violent sadomasochistic relationship.

My supervisor cautioned me to be alert to the developing transference. "He'll need to act out an abusive situation," she said. "Try not to fall into being the aggressor."

I didn't know exactly what to look for. Then one day my patient arrived for his appointment and told me he was thinking seriously of killing himself. He refused to consider checking himself into the hospital.

"I can't let you go," I said. "You're at risk."

"I'm leaving. You don't care whether I kill myself, anyhow," he said, starting for the door.

I called security, and the guards, the patient and I walked from the clinic to the emergency room. Once there, however, the patient became threatening and required restraints.

It wasn't until I was summarizing the case for my supervisor that I realized I had been maneuvered into helping to detain and restrain a patient struggling to leave a sadomasochistic relationship, just as an aggressor would. He left therapy instead.

"He's better at this than you are," my supervisor encouraged me. "He's been at it longer." In retrospect, we decided I might have been able to head off the problem by talking about it with him in advance, and, failing that, having a colleague accompany him to the emergency room.

I try to ride the crest of the transference, to point out to the patient when I feel these connections building, lest the wave crash and drown both of us. And I am told that my equilibrium has not been put to the real test. The once- or twice-a-week therapy I offer rarely spawns the raging tides of transference that come in the context of near-daily psychoanalysis. Psychiatrists have nicknamed that force "transference with a capital T."

The irrational connections flow both ways. When I feel them toward patients, they are called countertransference. I come to the clinic with my own life history, my own buried conflicts. There is the danger that I will play those issues out in the context of the therapy—unconsciously writing a script that the patient must act out.

When an older female outpatient of mine considered terminating therapy, for example, it occurred to me that she might be reacting to her son's moving away from home by severing our relationship. Before exploring that possibility, however, I needed to look at my own feelings. Was my desire to keep the patient in therapy rooted in my intense childhood fear of separation from my mother?

The pushes and pulls of transference and countertransference are much of the reason that some forms of psychotherapy rely on maintaining rigid structure to the therapeutic relationship. Visits are generally 50 minutes long. They take place in the office. They occur on a regular schedule. Their cost is fixed. The personal life of the therapist may be kept wholly out of the discussion. The doctor's home phone number may be withheld. Any variable introduced into the relationship without consideration may be a contaminant reflecting the unconscious wishes, needs and fears of either patient or doctor.

A patient who consistently talks past the end of the session, for example, may have a need to exert control. A therapist who gives no real notice of an upcoming vacation may be expressing anger or ambivalence about his or her role as a caregiver.

Even knowing all this, part of me would like to stop acting and become the lost son, trustworthy father, reliable friend or steadfast lover that my patients need or want. I fantasize that doing so would alleviate their pain. But that would mean abandoning the role I promised to play at the outset—that of an impartial and empathic observer. It would obliterate a valuable opportunity to demonstrate how the integrity of a relationship can be preserved.

As inadequate a remedy as it sometimes feels, therapy must remain a lens to bring life into focus, not a substitute for living.

The complexity of the therapist-patient relationship may sound imposing. Why would anyone sit for 50 minutes in a room with the frightened, angry, captivating ghosts of relationships long past?

The reason is that unresolved issues can cause the greatest damage under cover. We all walk an emotional minefield every day, with the explosives and treasures of the past spread everywhere before us. Psychotherapy at least begins to clarify the landscape.

5

Electroshock

The only solid piece of scientific truth about which I feel totally confident is that we are profoundly ignorant about nature. . . . It is this sudden confrontation with the depth and scope of ignorance that represents the most significant contribution of twentieth-century science to the human intellect.

Lewis Thomas   *The Medusa and the Snail*

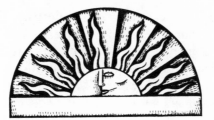

I'm not sure if I'm supposed to admit it as a psychiatrist in training, but electroconvulsive therapy—shock treatment—makes me nervous.

Like a lot of people, I remember vivid images of the practice from the movie *One Flew Over The Cuckoo's Nest*, but those aren't what I find discomforting. Advances in electroconvulsive therapy (ECT) have made the procedure more routine than startling. ECT has been proven to be remarkably effective against depression. I think I'm nervous because passing a small amount of electrical current through the brain does help alleviate some serious cases of depression, but for reasons no one can explain.

Not knowing how ECT works is hard for me to tolerate; as someone who has spent 11 years immersed in the study of science and medicine, I want to know precisely which gears of illness I interfere with. Strange that I worry little about the brain chemicals I set in motion with psychotherapy. I'm comfortable with intuition and insight. I'm a mind doctor. But when I use a machine and resort to electricity, I feel like a brain doctor. I wear my white coat. I drape a stethoscope around my neck.

The room is quiet. We talk softly. There is a box that looks like a small generator, maybe a foot square, with buttons and dials on it, a few wires protruding. A specialist administers general anesthesia, as well as a medicine that temporarily paralyzes all of the patient's muscles. This

29

prevents the violent convulsions that used to be caused by more primitive forms of shock treatment.

In order to know that modern ECT is working at all, we inflate a blood pressure cuff on one arm. That stops the paralyzing medicine from circulating to it, and that arm is the only part of the body that moves during the seizure. We need to see something move because the seizure tells us that the ECT is causing a major electrical disturbance in the brain, and longer seizures mean a more effective treatment.

The electrodes are half-dollar–sized metal plates covered with conductive gel. Typically, one is held firmly to the patient's temple and another to the top of his or her head. With the patient asleep, a button is pressed to deliver a two-second dose of electricity. There is no frightening noise, no wild jerking, no pain. Attention focuses on that one arm as it bends stiffly at the elbow and shakes. We clock the time, ideally 30 to 60 seconds, until it relaxes. It may be only minutes before the patient leaves the room, awake and moving.

That, anticlimactic as it may sound, is high drama for psychiatrists. Many of us don't think of ourselves as doing things to patients. Not in the way a surgeon thinks of cutting out a clogged length of artery. We are trained in diligence and patience. We accept that the fruits of our labor may be a delicate change in perspective or rise in self-esteem. Even when we use medicines, we know that improvement may take weeks or months. We learn to accept subtle recoveries. A seizure as evidence of our intervention stands in sharp contrast to our usual slow and cautious approach.

The fact is that ECT works better than counseling or medication for some patients. Some studies have shown that as many as 90 percent of drug-resistant depressed patients improved, generally with 6 to 12 treatments. Because depression is often an episodic illness and the effect of ECT doesn't last forever, it may need to be repeated.

There are theories about why ECT works. Causing a major electrical disturbance in the brain may help fight depression by exhausting more random, abnormal discharges. Or it may work because it increases or diminishes the sensitivity of various chemical receptors in the brain. These receptors receive messages via the same chemical messengers in the brain that are disordered in people who are suffering from depression.

Why, if ECT is so effective, do we use it so infrequently? One reason is that the procedure carries the complications and risks of general anesthesia, with approximately one death in every 25,000 cases. Another is that ECT can cause loss of memory, particularly of events that occur just prior to treatment. Although the amnesia is usually mild and, in fact, undetectable after several months, some patients complain of lasting memory problems.

Medicines, of course, have their own side effects. And, sometimes, these are more alarming than the ones associated with ECT.

The real reasons have more to do with fear than facts. ECT has a bad reputation, a legacy of the decades when it was used indiscriminately without anesthesia and towels were stuffed in the mouths of patients to prevent them from biting off their tongues. In those circumstances, bones sometimes fractured from the force of muscle contractions.

Hollywood, as in *Cuckoo's Nest*, did its part by portraying ECT as a way of punishing free thinkers and controlling their minds. It is no surprise that, to this day, those who benefit from the treatment are reluctant to support it publicly, lest they be branded defective or incompetent.

Unlike medications, ECT is not profitable to industry. If it were, there might be a flurry of industry-supported research to document its effectiveness and reduce its stigma. Psychiatrists would get the same hard-sell educational materials on ECT as we do on antidepressants. Maybe even some pens, pads of paper and briefcases with little lightning bolts or something, just like the ones we get with drug logos. But it's the power company that is paid for electrical current, not a pharmaceutical manufacturer.

Doctors make decisions in a complex social context. We incorporate in our treatments the acceptability—to ourselves, the patient, the public and the profession—of the therapeutic strategies we employ. And the fact is that psychiatrists remain more reluctant to perform ECT than to use many medications that can have more lasting side effects.

So it may be that, even when ECT would be the most effective treatment for a patient, it won't be prescribed. Not because it won't work, but because it won't be well received.

6

What Kind of Cure?

The desire to take medicine is perhaps the greatest feature which distinguishes man from animals.

Sir William Osler *Science and Immorality*

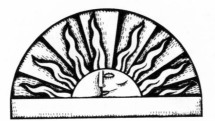

L ost in the controversy over whether Prozac increases suicidal thoughts in some patients is an issue of even greater significance for psychiatry and society. When does a medicine cease being a treatment for disease and become a cure-all for unhappiness?

Prozac has captured the American psyche in a way no antidepressant ever has. It is effective—for short periods of time—for people diagnosed with severe depression, a major mental illness with specific signs and symptoms. But now, it is also being used as a more general remedy for despondency and as a substitute for psychotherapy.

Discouraged patients who suffer no major mental illness are, nonetheless, requesting to be treated with Prozac. Some family physicians are prescribing it liberally for patients who complain of persistent unhappiness. Friends of mine have half-jokingly asked whether I can get them samples. They wonder aloud if they might not think "better" with the drug than they do without it, that perhaps they are "missing something."

Prozac, the brand name of the drug fluoxetine, is one of a new generation of antidepressants thought to work primarily by enhancing a brain chemical messenger called serotonin. Since it was approved by the Food and Drug Administration in 1987, it has become the antidepressant most widely prescribed by psychiatrists in America.

I have found Prozac very useful in treating depression. The drug's broad appeal may even help to diminish the stigma associated with

35

receiving psychiatric treatment. But history tells us to be wary when a psychiatric drug achieves popularity.

Valium, for example, had its own honeymoon period. It seemed to relieve a wide range of mental distress without significant side effects. Only later was the degree of its addictive potential appreciated.

The public debate on Prozac—which has ranged from court hearings to an FDA panel—centers on whether the drug can trigger violent actions by users. A few patients have said that Prozac induced them to commit murder. Doctors and mental health experts agree, however, that used and monitored properly, Prozac is an important therapeutic tool.

While Prozac may never show any other side effect than it has to date, the level of public applause for the drug makes me uncomfortable.

Colleagues tell me that some of their patients who take Prozac report feeling as if they have completely new brains. Some patients are reluctant to decrease or stop the medication, even after several months or a year of treatment with it. While extended usage is commonplace, the Prozac package insert reads:

The effectiveness of Prozac in long-term use, that is, for more than five to six weeks, has not been systematically evaluated in controlled trials. Therefore, the physician who elects to use Prozac for extended periods should periodically reevaluate the long-term usefulness of the drug for the individual patient.

The insert also states:

Prozac has not been systematically studied, in animals or humans, for its potential for abuse, tolerance or physical dependence.

In other words, no formal testing has ruled out the possibility that long-term use of Prozac could be either psychologically or physically addictive.

But Prozac's unknown long-term side effects are not my sole concern. More worrisome to me, Prozac seems to be perceived by some as a substitute for insight-oriented psychotherapy, a shortcut to the benefits of knowing oneself, what psychoanalysts call an examined life.

Two of the psychiatry residents I questioned about their experience prescribing Prozac surprised me with the response, "I take it. And it certainly works for me." Each added, "It's a lot cheaper than analysis."

Free samples of Prozac are distributed to physicians in little boxes that contain seven 20-milligram tablets. The boxes are labeled "ONE WEEK'S THERAPY," rather than one week's supply or one week's treatment.

But Prozac isn't psychotherapy in a box. It is an effective medicine for treating some cases of major depression, but it can't offer the same self-knowledge and self-possession that come with understanding the psychological dynamics at work in one's life.

Recently, a middle-aged man, on whose case I was consulting, confided in me that he was planning to stop his psychotherapy. He and his therapist had been meeting weekly for several years. Together, they had confronted his painful memories of being physically abused as a child and had tried to understand and control his involvement in drugs and crime as an adult.

He credited the relationship with allowing him to develop personal insights that had tempered his anger. It had also been his sole support during his divorce and the period of homelessness that followed. Then, during a hospital admission for alcohol treatment three months before our meeting, he had complained of low mood and insomnia and been started on Prozac.

His symptoms improved with the drug, but his decision to stop seeing his therapist surprised me.

"Why are you considering ending therapy now?" I asked.

"I'm just not getting anything out of it," he said. "Ever since the Prozac, I don't feel things the way I used to. I can talk about being abused when I was a kid, and it's just an everyday discussion. It might as well have happened to someone else."

"You are less depressed, though . . . Right?" I asked.

He pondered the question. "I am less depressed," he said, shrugging his shoulders. "I've got the same problems, but they're buried."

I have heard similar descriptions from other patients. They feel less sad after receiving Prozac but complain that real contentment remains elusive and that the road to achieving it seems blocked.

To invoke a vision of a Brave New World, in which mental distress is no longer a cause for reflection, but simply cause for a prescription, may seem alarmist. But psychiatry, which should have been a natural ally of the examined life, has seemed oddly embarrassed to speak forcefully for it. Professionals in the field have watched rather passively as the pharmaceutical, managed care, and insurance industries have lined up in support of quick (and incomplete) fixes for psychiatric distress.

The work of interpersonal understanding, used in conjunction with medications as needed, is a more arduous, often more expensive and time-consuming road, recommended chiefly by the fact that patients feel it leads somewhere.

7

Ranging Far
From Reality

Hope is a waking dream.

Aristotle *Lives of Eminent Philosophers*

The growth of the mind is the widening of the range of
consciousness, and . . . each step forward has been a most
painful and laborious achievement.

Jung *Contributions to Analytical Psychology*

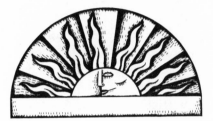

The devastation that comes with psychiatric illness may obscure mental potential of equal magnitude. Disorders of thought and perception that cause patients extreme distress hint at enormous untapped creativity of the mind. What if thinking patterns related to psychosis could be refined by medical intervention or natural evolution and allow our minds to safely range far from reality?

A man I recently treated had lost his wife in tragic circumstances some years before. When his daughter revealed plans to move out of state, her impending departure seemed too much to bear. The daughter he knew would never be so callous. He became convinced that she had been kidnapped and that the person threatening to abandon him was a masquerading double.

The differences between the two young women, he asserted, were subtle but unmistakable. His real daughter's hair was finer than that of the double who now claimed her place. Her nose had been angled slightly more to the right.

My patient was so convinced of the abduction that he had filed a missing person's report with the police and had contacted the FBI. It was obvious to him, however, that no one was taking his concern seriously. He felt utterly alone against an awesome enemy capable of assuming any human form it chose.

The terrifying condition with which my patient was grappling has been called Capgras' syndrome, named for the French psychiatrist Jean Marie Joseph Capgras. It is generally the hallmark of an underlying major mental illness, such as schizophrenia, depression or mania. The main symptom of the syndrome is the patient's false and unshakable belief (called a *delusion*) that other individuals in his or her life are not their real selves, but imposters, often with evil intent. Some psychiatrists have theorized that the evil double thus created is the mind's way of banishing a loved one's negative qualities, allowing the patient to maintain an ideal image of that person.

Capgras' syndrome clearly represents disordered thinking and brings with it intense emotional distress. But perhaps a massive, unrealized creativity of the human mind is reflected in such psychosis.

The fact that an individual can dramatically recast characters in his or her life story is at once frightening and paradoxically hopeful. It speaks to the mind's ability to recreate an alternate vision of the world and to free us from painful realities. It also hints at the promise of closer connections between human beings. If the mind can exorcise an unwieldy daughter, could it be called upon to turn a stranger into a family member?

In a way, mental illness may be like immunological disease. In most cases of Addison's disease, for example, the immune system—our intricate line of defense against infection—has been misdirected, responding to the adrenal gland as a foreign invader. The resulting destruction of the adrenal gland depletes the body of vital hormones and can cause symptoms including muscle cramps, fainting, vomiting, coma and death.

Were we limited to a snapshot of these traitorous antibodies assaulting the adrenal gland, visiting such pain and suffering, we might see the immune system as a pure enemy. We would miss its marvelous ability to insulate the body and allow us to walk freely amidst bacteria and viruses that would otherwise cut us down.

Capgras' syndrome is just one example of the mind turned on itself. Often, on the medical and surgical wards to which I consult, patients who have lapsed into the confusion and disorientation of delirium report hearing the voices of, or actually seeing, loved ones who are nowhere nearby. Their impaired perceptions are caused by bodily abnormalities, such as widespread infection or too little oxygen to the brain.

Yet these cases also testify to a kind of mental agility. At a time of biological and psychological stress, the brain has summoned convincing representations of important figures in the patient's life. If these frightening experiences can be born of physiology gone awry, perhaps other changes in that same physiology could lead toward an ability to bring more comforting memories to life.

Even outside the realm of delusions and hallucinations, psychiatric symptoms often seem woven of both pain and poetry. A grandmother I treated had been referred to me for a constant burning sensation in her feet. A team of doctors, including a vascular surgeon and a neurologist, had searched for an abnormality that could explain her suffering. They had measured the blood flow to her feet and tested the nerves and muscles. They had analyzed her blood chemistry, searching for the uric acid of gout or the sugar of diabetes. They had even imaged the base of her spine, where nerves serving the feet originate, to make sure that no tumor or deformity of bone was interfering with these nerves. They could find no explanation.

As if to say that words would fail her, she took off her ankle boots and socks moments after sitting down in my office. "Look how red they are," she said. "Like fire."

I examined her feet, which seemed perfectly normal. "How long has the pain lasted?" I asked.

"Two months, already," she said tearfully. "And no doctor can tell me what's wrong. They think it's in my head."

It wasn't until the end of our second session that my patient briefly mentioned her grandson, who was serving with the military in Saudi Arabia.

"Saudi Arabia? How long has he been there?" I asked.

"Oh, about two months, I guess."

"Has he written you what it's like?"

"It's a desert," she said. She shrugged. "Hot sand everywhere."

My patient turned out to be suffering from depression. Her pain was only one symptom of that condition. But it was also an expression of her particular life story, an unconscious response to her grandson's experience and testimony to the potential of human empathy. If a grandmother's feet can burn with the heat off sand thousands of miles away, might all of us one day empathize with others far away by experiencing their suffering?

All these observations, of course, are grounded at least as much in philosophy as science. Still, it seems possible to me that some forms of psychiatric illness may represent a way station in the evolution of the mind.

Perhaps we are just seeing another snapshot in which neurobiology is flexing its muscles, causing terrible growing pains as human beings slowly develop valuable new patterns of thought and perception.

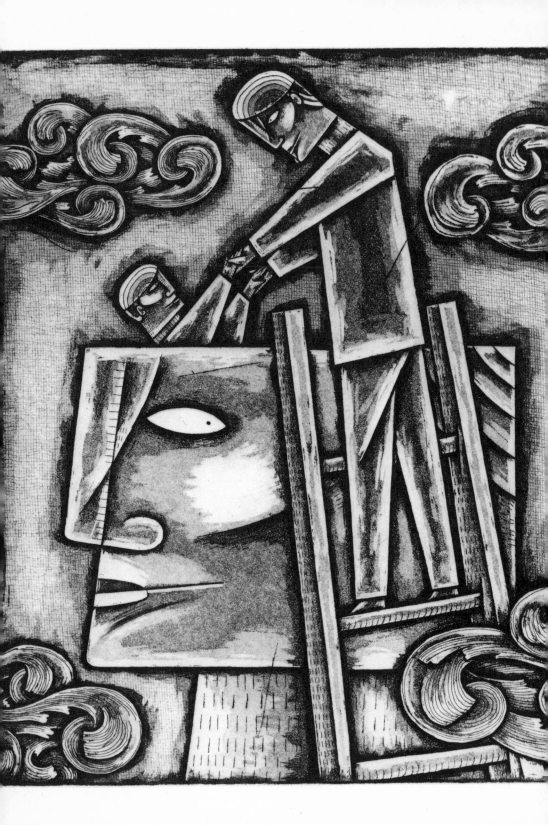

An Examined Life

8

Reaping the Benefits of an Examined Life

Physician, heal thyself.

Luke 4:23

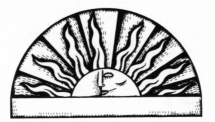

*I*n medical school, when I first considered becoming a psychiatrist, one of my mentors, an eye surgeon, assured me I wasn't the type. "People go into that field because they have problems of their own to work out," he said.

His warning disturbed me. I don't believe I was particularly bothered by the implication that psychiatrists were emotional misfits: I knew some, and they didn't seem to be. I also wasn't surprised that the stigma borne by psychiatric patients would extend to those who worked with them.

What bothered me was the idea that psychiatrists would enter the field in order to treat themselves, which seemed like a violation of the model of a helping profession. It cast them as hybrid doctor-patients, taking while giving.

My worry over this, together with my interest in psychiatric medications, resulted in a knee-jerk reaction against psychiatrists who were undergoing psychotherapy or psychoanalysis. Once the rule, being in therapy is now an option only half the psychiatrists-in-training I know have chosen. To me, they seemed not to understand which side of the stethoscope they were supposed to be on.

But after three years of residency, I now know that the surgeon may have sensed one of the crucial elements of practicing psychiatry and either feared or misunderstood it.

Psychiatrists do focus on their own emotional development and growth. Many of us, having learned the role of the unconscious in shaping present behavior, don't want to live at the mercy of such forces. But, at least as important, we know that avoiding these issues in our own lives can diminish the clarity with which we view the lives of our patients.

It is an essential part of my job to be aware of how my personal history might affect my response to hearing a patient's story. If, for example, I feel anxious during psychotherapy, I try to understand why. I wonder if the patient is speaking about something that echoes an experience or conflict of my own. I may detect that his or her tone of voice and mannerisms remind me of someone else I feel strongly about. I may review my day, looking for remnants of events that are contaminating the current hour.

Recognizing these transplanted emotions and their roots helps to prevent them from silently directing therapy, discouraging my exploration of one theme in the patient's life while encouraging my interest in another. A by-product of this internal editing is a kind of self analysis. In attempting to understand my emotional responses to patients, I reap some of the benefits of an examined life.

One man I treated, for example, began each of his jobs by warning his supervisors that he had no intention of fitting any rigid mold they envisioned for him. He made it clear that he was unpredictable. On those occasions when his employers reacted by excluding him from their projects, however, he felt misunderstood and hurt.

From childhood, he had been pushed to enter his successful father's profession but had refused. "I always wondered whether he loved me in spite of it," he said.

I was immediately moved by his story. I understood how his desire to be unconditionally accepted by his father had prompted his paradoxical distancing from—and yearning for acceptance by—other male authority figures in his life.

In wondering why I felt a sense of camaraderie pursuing this theme with him, I realized that my patient's unconscious tug-of-war with supervisors could describe some of my own experiences.

As a young man, I had worried whether my parents would lose respect for me if I abandoned my plans to study medicine.

I hadn't been able to put this dynamic into words until my patient did. The context of helping another person understand his life made it possible—and necessary—for me to understand part of mine.

It has taken me the better part of my training to integrate this introspection with my notion of a healer. In other specialties, the doctor's presumed vigor in the face of the patient's sickness adds to the professional's position of power. A sense of invulnerability can develop, which is sometimes comforting to those working amidst tragedy. Becoming a psychotherapist requires surrendering much of that distance. We come to our work as human beings. We are vulnerable. We resonate with the stories we hear. In service to patients, we regularly turn our "stethoscopes" on ourselves.

This can be a particularly stressful brand of reflection. Seeing oneself in the conflicts of a troubled or ill person can require revisiting painful events that have been relegated to the unconscious. Long-forgotten emotions can be awakened unexpectedly.

I do not, in the context of performing psychotherapy, get these discoveries off my chest. Even when I feel the impulse to share my personal experiences, I must keep them to myself and use them only to focus the patient's exploration of his or her life.

In trying to help a middle-aged patient cope with disabilities caused by his stroke, for example, I noted how uneasy his story made me. "It came out of the blue," he said. "I never had any symptoms, never smoked, never had high blood pressure, nothing."

It was a few days before I related my anxiety about working with him directly to my own dread of sudden, catastrophic injury or illness. I found some of the childhood basis for that fear in my father's narrow escape from a deadly train crash, my mother's unexpected, life-threatening surgery, and a childhood friend who was diagnosed with cancer.

"I can see how terrifying it is to think this could happen without warning . . . or that it could happen again," I said later. My patient nodded, his eyes welling with tears.

What I hadn't mentioned was my fear that it could happen to me or to someone I love. I took those feelings home.

The bits and pieces of personal insight that flow to the therapist can be unwieldy. In trying to make sense of my own life, I find myself sharing fresh memories of old, often unspoken conflicts with friends and relatives. They are not always emotionally prepared to reflect on the issues I have uncovered and sometimes react with distance or anger.

"Why are you rehashing ancient history?" a relative complained recently. "Are you trying to start trouble?"

The stress of self-discovery is another reason psychiatrists them-

selves enter therapy or analysis. A colleague can provide a safe environment in which to explore the personal questions that practicing psychiatry raises.

Although it has been suggested by my supervisors, I have not begun
this process myself. Not long ago, I would have seen my avoidance of
the patient's role as evidence of strength and professionalism. Now I see
it as something to overcome.

9

Personal Connections

It strikes me—what are these sudden fits of complete exhaustion? I come in here to write; can't even finish a sentence; and am pulled under; now is this some odd effort; the subconscious pulling me down into her? . . . No. I think the effort to live in two spheres: the novel and life; is a strain. . . . To have to behave with circumspection and decision to strangers wrenches me into another region; hence the collapse.

Virginia Woolf

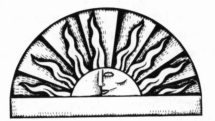

A patient of mine, who first sought psychiatric care after her son's unexpected death, recently paged me at the hospital. She tearfully explained that her grandchild had died the previous day and that she would be missing our appointment in order to attend the funeral.

I had met with her more than 50 times, seen her through the terrifying psychosis fueled by her first loss, listened to the torments of her childhood and failed marriage. This new tragedy took me by surprise. I was saddened, but I was also frustrated and angry that my patient's hard-won emotional equilibrium should again be threatened by something so random and seemingly unfair as another untimely death.

"I'm so sorry," was all I could say.

"I know," she said. "If I need to call, I will. Otherwise, I'll be in to see you next week."

As we said goodbye, an unexpected emotion was already mingling with my sadness and anger. I felt isolated. I had been privy to intimate details of my patient's family life. I had been moved by her closely held belief that this grandchild magically reflected her deceased son.

Part of me felt I belonged at that funeral, that I should have the opportunity not only to pay my respects, but also to mourn. Yet the therapist-patient relationship, appropriately framed by the clinic walls, left me alone with my feelings.

I have, for years now, been storing away bits of joy and worry and pride and despair—the fruit of emotional connections I have been privileged to make with patients. It has been easy to contain each one, but their cumulative weight is more unwieldy. I feel as if a library of my patients' penetrating stories are loose inside me.

The dynamics of therapy make me a temporary central character in dozens of such dramas. Through the forces of transference and counter-transference, patient and therapist invest each other with qualities that actually belong to other important figures in their lives.

At certain moments, I realize that patients are responding to me as they would to a son, brother, father or lover.

I often notice I have warmed to these roles. A woman I have treated for two years, for example, recently became engaged. In asking about her fiancé, I realized that our discussion closely resembled one a father might have with his daughter. My physicianly concern was flirting with fatherly concern.

These irrational connections are expected by-products of the therapeutic process. By identifying and exploring them, psychiatrists hope that patients will come to better understand the real relationships from which they are derived.

What seems to be weighing on me is that these irrational connections tap real, not phantom, emotion. When I uncover and explain them, the parts of me invested in them die. Working amidst such forces sometimes feels like struggling through endless vines that brush against me, then pull me here and there, only to break unpredictably.

Relationships with patients I have come to care about can end without notice and without ceremony. One inpatient I treated took his own life months after I rotated to another hospital. I heard of his death, in passing, a week after it occurred.

Another patient I worked closely with for a year lost his job and left treatment. He had been struggling to heal the scars of a traumatic childhood and to overcome drug addiction. I have not heard from him since.

When I take overnight shifts covering the state hospital where I used to work full time, I exchange mere greetings with patients who have touched me deeply.

This distance is, of course, necessary. The effectiveness of therapy is partly dependent on its structure. I am speaking only of the personal toll—the occult emotional bleed—from being the cloistered repository for piercing fragments of so many lives.

Outside the hospital, I have become reluctant to squeeze another story inside me. My connections with patients and the depth of the issues they address lead me to expect similar intensity from friends and family. Their voices need to be more urgent than ever to move me.

Upon hearing from my father that an acquaintance of our family was sick, I found myself immediately seeking to establish how sick. Once I learned the illness wasn't very threatening, it was difficult for me to listen.

Even when the subjects friends and family raise are powerful, the therapeutic distance I have refined can persist. At times, I hear compliments, criticism and even expressions of love as a third party might. It is as if entering and exiting so many compelling life stories is beginning to allow me to enter and exit my own.

This distance may be a kind of defense. The unpredictable nature of my connections with patients makes me reflect on the fragility of my personal relationships. If I can be treated (and even respond) as a patient's brother one day, only to rotate to another hospital and never return, how indestructible is my relationship with my sister? If evanescent fathers and mothers can parade in and out of my office, how sturdy are my connections to my parents?

These little, pseudo deaths are making me dwell on real impending losses. In a kind of surrender to the impermanence of relationships, I fear I am preemptively detaching from people I have cherished. It may be no accident that the past months have seen me sever a close friendship, a four-year-long romantic relationship and a nine-year-long business relationship.

The highest poetry in this may be that the source of these dynamics—the cognitive changes wrought by psychiatry training—is also my best hope for understanding and harnessing them. Helping others come to terms with their loves and losses will always, I now see, require coming to terms with my own.

10

Ambivalence

I feel more confident and more satisfied when I reflect that I have two professions and not one. Medicine is my lawful wife and literature is my mistress. When I get tired of one I spend the night with the other. Though it's disorderly it's not so dull, and besides, neither really loses anything through my infidelity.

Anton Pavlovich Chekhov, September 11, 1888,
Letter to A. S. Suvorin

I would like to be a free artist and nothing else, and I regret God has not given me the strength to be one.

Anton Pavlovich Chekhov, October 4, 1888,
Letter to Alexi Pleshcheev

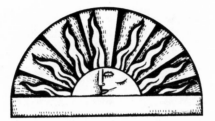

*E*very week I meet with about a dozen other psychiatrists-in-training, led by an older therapist, to talk about patients. Each of us must present a patient's psychiatric history to the group. This is an imposing task, because the group has become expert in deciphering which issues in the therapist's own life might be reflected in the patient he or she has chosen.

This essay began as my presentation to the group. My fellow psychiatry residents may well resent my sharing it with you. Why, they might wonder, must I let readers in on this private medical discussion?

The reason is that I serve two Muses—one presiding over psychiatry and the other over writing. In spending time exclusively with one, I worry the other might leave on grounds of neglect. And this would be, for me, a kind of death.

I know that inviting you into the group—even vicariously—is close to a violation of the rules. It is, to borrow from Chekhov, the unabashed introduction of my mistress to my wife, complete with the extraordinary hope that the two might begin a dialogue and even become fast friends.

The patient I presented was a 47-year-old homeless white man, with a history of a stroke five years before. He had been admitted after coming to the emergency room drunk and suicidal, with a very high blood alcohol level. His vague chief complaint was that he had not been the same since the bleeding in his brain.

But that summary, with its emphasis on data and symptoms, risks missing important parts of the person. It wouldn't satisfy a reader's need to understand the inner workings of a character, and it shouldn't satisfy a conscientious physician's need to understand a patient.

What struck me first about the patient was that he looked like a pudgy, but obviously powerful 47-year-old boy with a crew cut. He spoke quietly, seemingly without emotion, even when talking about pain or love. He told me he was depressed and anxious and couldn't sleep because of nightmares. He didn't feel like eating. The only visible hint of despair came when he mentioned that his girlfriend had started to insist that he propose marriage.

But was the hint of pain I thought I saw in my patient's face my own invention? Was it his fear of commitment to one woman, or the reflection of my own? And why should such musings feel like an interruption in his case history, rather than the very heart of it?

The next step in the presentation usually is a checklist of symptoms revealed through observation and direct questioning.

The patient was neither homicidal nor paranoid. He denied experiencing any hallucinations. He was alert and knew the date and the name of the hospital. His concentration was not impaired, his attention span was normal and his memory was intact.

Next comes the patient's past history. My patient had started drinking as a youngster. He stole his first beer from a store and still remembers the alcohol making him feel fearless, like a gangster. He drank more and more throughout his teens, up to a case a day.

During the early 1960s, he first experienced what he called "wild anxiety." Although he didn't relate the two, the anxiety happened to start when he proposed to a woman he'd met in college. All of a sudden he couldn't work, sleep or eat. He left the woman, increased his drinking and started hearing voices that told him to kill himself. The voices went away after he spent a few weeks alone.

Then, following another failed relationship in the mid-1980s, the right side of his thalamus, a part of the brain that plays a major role in regulating emotion, started to bleed.

The scientist in me knows the questions raised by that stroke. Did my patient suffer high blood pressue? Had an aneurism burst? Were the arteries and veins in his brain malformed since birth?

But is it folly for the poet in me to wonder first about a connection between lost loves and stroke, about emotions disrupting anatomy? Why dismiss my quiet suspicion that this patient's conflicted emotional state could have worked his thalamus into such a frenzy that the little blood vessels supplying it burst?

Strange that I feel more confident presenting the fact that my patient's CT scan showed the brain pressed to one side in his skull and that he experienced difficulty walking, which gradually improved.

The family history is next in the formal presentation. My patient didn't trust his father, an abusive man who drank excessively and frequently left home in the middle of the night.

"Where was he going?" I once asked.

"I don't know."

"Did he work nights?"

"Who knows? Maybe he had a woman," my patient said. "So what?"

I let the issue drop.

I should have asked much more about it. I also should have asked more about my patient's mother and the women he had left. I should have ferreted out how his new girlfriend's desire for a commitment was related to his current symptoms. But I was much newer at treating patients than I am now. I was caught up in the technical scientific debate over whether the patient had bipolar or unipolar affective disorder and whether to prescribe the antidepressant fluoxetine or desipramine. I wasn't seeing the patient whole.

I eventually prescribed both drugs because sometimes the two fight depression better than either alone. And, in about three weeks, my patient seemed less sad. He had stopped talking about killing himself. He was sleeping and eating. But he still kept saying, "It's like I have this spot inside me that I'd like to rub, 'cause it hurts, but I can't get at it." I wrote that down for possible use in an essay—and increased the fluoxetine.

I don't think that spot ever really left him. Maybe it had something to do with his father's philandering. Maybe that unconscious lesson had partly set my patient up to run from women who might, otherwise, have had his complete allegiance.

That fear—being consumed by a single passion—is one I share with my patient. Although I have two Muses, I have one love. The truth is that my Muses turn out not only to be friends, but chambers of the same heart. I suspect Chekhov's wife and mistress were also one passion. Each individual's illness is a unique drama, and every good physician must be, in some measure, a storyteller.

11

The Last Night On Call

In a real dark night of the soul it is always three o'clock in the morning.

F. Scott Fitzgerald "The Crack-up"

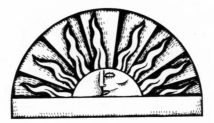

When I saw a person through the chicken wire–reinforced glass of the observation window, I felt the dread that descends whenever psychiatry night call begins with a patient already waiting in the emergency room.

I'd just come from a full day's work at the Boston Veterans Administration Hospital and had hoped for some rest before beginning the next 15-hour shift at New England Medical Center. That hope, I reminded myself, had probably doomed me to no sleep at all; it is a superstition of residents that anticipating a slow night guarantees a busy one.

"Taking call" is the defining burden of residency, the aspect of training that feels most like servitude to the hospital and least like education. The job involves sometimes sleepless 15- or 24-hour shifts, helping people who need everything from simple reassurance to emergency hospitalization.

Being on call forces me to contain my frustration with the complicated, unpredictable nature of the work and to quell the anxiety aroused by the loneliness that can set in after midnight when the rest of the world seems to be asleep.

Yet on this, my last of more than 200 required nights on call, I felt nostalgia mixing with a sense of liberation. I have treated patients in the midst of flashbacks to war atrocities, depressed patients who have made near-fatal suicide attempts, teenagers facing terrifying first episodes of psychosis, patients so paranoid that they refused to speak, and others so fearful of what imaginary voices were saying that they begged to be placed in leather restraints.

I walked to the glass-enclosed office in the center of the emergency room and glanced at the schedule on the wall. It was not our turn to serve as the admitting facility for homeless, mentally ill patients.

"It shouldn't be too bad," said a colleague, nodding at the waiting patient. "She's probably going to be a voluntary admission to our ward. Also, the weather's nice." Another residents' theory: mild weather means fewer ER patients.

Walking to the call room, I felt a little relief. I still had to write up the patient's history and perform a physical examination, but it was an advantage that our ward was agreeing to admit her. Otherwise, it might take hours to present the case to as many as a dozen hospitals in an effort to find an available bed that matched her insurance.

I dumped my overnight bag in the 7-foot by 8-foot–sized call room and, remembering recent thefts, covered the bag with a sheet. The room was grim and humid: a water pipe was being repaired, which had left a gaping hole and small flying insects clinging to the walls.

I walked into the examining room and greeted the patient, a middle-aged woman. Hours earlier, she had expressed serious suicidal thoughts to her therapist. My impulse was to get her quickly to the inpatient unit upstairs. Not knowing when more patients might arrive, I always worked with a sense of urgency.

"I'm going to try to help make your admission here go smoothly," I said.

"I think I'd rather go home," she replied, uneasily pacing back and forth. "I'll be fine."

That simple statement threatened hours of work. If she refused to stay, I would have to evaluate whether she was potentially suicidal enough to warrant involuntary hospitalization. If I concluded that she was, and she tried to leave, I would have to restrain or medicate her against her will. Our unlocked psychiatric unit would then no longer be appropriate for her. I would have to search for a bed on a locked ward.

I sat down, facing her, with the goal of making her more comfortable with the idea of hospitalization. "We haven't met before," I said, "but I know your therapist is very concerned about you . . . Tell me in your own words what's been happening in your life."

She readily told me how exhausted and overwhelmed she felt as a single parent caring for a disabled child. Weeping, she agreed to hospitalization.

While she was telling me that she didn't need to be on a locked ward, I noticed a second patient being escorted to an examination room. I quickly finished the interview, assigned a medical student to do the required physical examination and prepared to greet the next patient.

Just then my beeper alerted me to a phone call from outside the hospital. Being on call also means taking phone calls that come into the hospital's main switchboard from anyone with after-hours concerns related to psychiatry. These range from simple questions about medication side effects to pleas for help to resist suicidal or homicidal impulses. Sometimes, I have had to send the police to the caller's address to bring him or her to the emergency room for evaluation.

"I feel like jumping out of my skin," said a male voice.

"Can you tell me a little bit more about how you're feeling?" I asked.

"I'm not coming in there. You'll admit me."

"I'd really just like to know how you're—" I began. The man hung up.

I wondered whether he would eventually arrive at the emergency room. Part of me hoped he would come for help, another part of me worried about getting backed up with patients. The frustration and uncertainty of a long wait can make potentially violent patients lose control.

The second patient had come with her husband. Her symptoms were largely physical—nausea and severe headache—but the couple assured me they were typical for her anxiety disorder. She had suffered many years of similar distress, often brought on by family discord, and had been admitted to another hospital with the same symptoms a few weeks earlier. As she described her aches and pains, I noticed that her husband was rolling his eyes.

"This must be wearing on both of you," I said. The woman began to cry. "I can't go on anymore," she said.

"I'm completely worn out," her husband muttered, shaking his head.

I had to make a quick assessment. I turned to her husband: "Are you feeling like not going on, too?"

After he assured me he was not depressed or suicidal, I concentrated on his wife. Since she could not guarantee that she would be able to resist killing herself, I knew she would have to be admitted somewhere. Although she had had physical symptoms for years, I still needed to make sure there was no new medical problem. As I was taking her history, a nurse opened the door and announced that a third patient, a male graduate student weeping uncontrollably, was waiting.

He told me that nothing specific had gone wrong, that his depression had come out of nowhere. "It feels like I'm receding, and the world is just going forward," he said. "All I want to do is die."

At midnight, after two hours spent arranging for him and the second patient to be admitted to other hospitals—luckily both had good insurance—I headed for a few hours' sleep in the call room. I chuckled as I recalled a relative asking why psychiatry residents needed to take overnight call. "What could possibly happen?" he wondered. "If someone's upset, can't it wait until morning?"

At 3 A.M., the intercom poised on a shelf over my bed blared that another patient had arrived in the emergency room. Swearing, I rubbed my eyes and fumbled for the light switch, reminding myself that the patient needed help and the nurse who called me was just doing her job. There was no one to be angry at. I shoved the intercom off the shelf and felt better.

The patient, a man in his forties, had arrived from the Midwest weeks earlier. Although he had a history of alcoholism, he insisted he had not had anything to drink. Normally, I would worry about withdrawal, but his vital signs were entirely normal. His chief complaint was that he had begun to hear imaginary voices, but he didn't know what they were saying.

"Tranquilizers—that Ativan stuff or Valium—makes them go away," he said.

I suspected he might be looking for drugs. "We try not to make a habit of giving out medicines from the emergency room," I said.

"Well, I have nowhere to sleep," he admitted.

Once he had convinced me he was not suicidal, I offered to call a nearby shelter and try to secure a bed. We were both relieved when one was available; he left 45 minutes later.

He was the last patient on my final overnight call. With his departure, my youth in psychiatry ended. In time, I hope to forget the lingering frustration of so many nights struggling to reconcile resentment and empathy.

12

Saying Goodbye
With Grace

I am a part of all that I have met . . .

Lord Tennyson

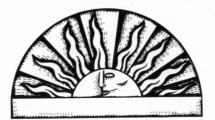

When will you be leaving, then?" my patient asked, her voice straining to remain composed, even kind.

"My work at this clinic ends in 10 weeks," I said. This part of my residency training was over; it was time to move on. I had met more than 80 times with this woman, a widow in her sixties. She had first come to see me two years earlier, suffering panic attacks and nightmares. These were the legacies of childhood brutalities inflicted by a sadistic brother. She was also grieving the loss of her husband, who had died a few years before, and her youngest son's move away from home. Slowly, a combination of psychotherapy and antianxiety medication had relieved most of her symptoms.

Now she looked more weary to me, more worn by adversity than at any time during our therapy. "I suppose I've known from the start you'd be leaving. What will you be doing?" she asked.

"I'll be working at the state hospital and writing," I said.

Suddenly, the news of my departure seemed to take hold. She stiffened. "Good," she said. Her face became a mixture of false courage and resentment. "Tell whomever's left that I'll be coming for my medicine once a month, period. No more of this once-a-week garbage. I don't think I ever needed to be here, in the first place."

I wanted to confess that I was worried about her, that I didn't want the end of our relationship to become another traumatic chapter in her life. But my role as a therapist was to continue helping her to overcome her fears about the inevitable losses in life. "I know my leaving is bound to bring up——," I began.

"Listen," she interrupted. She looked away. "I never told anyone my secrets before. They were mine. I'm not really sure why I told you. But I am certainly not going to share them with anyone else."

I heard a similar response from a successful business executive who had become depressed when his wife divorced him. He chuckled to himself as he listened to my plans. "So, you're blowing me off, like the old lady did," he said sarcastically. "Make sure I can get my Prozac refilled. That's all I'll need."

"We still have a few months to work together," I said to him.

"As far as I'm concerned, once you say you're leaving, you're gone," he shrugged. "I'm sure whatever you'll be doing has got to be better than listening to my sorry life story."

Leaving patients—terminating, to use the technical term—strips away any camouflage obscuring the fact that the doctor-patient relationship is at the heart of psychiatric treatment. The sadness, anger and fear that come with termination testify that real interpersonal bonds are being torn. With their emotional reactions, these and other patients reaffirmed my belief that therapy can never be reduced to prescription blanks.

The human connections that develop during psychotherapy are not only warm and supportive but also the raw material for insight that allows people to overcome problematic relationships.

Therapy serves as a theater of emotions into which patients unconsciously bring feelings transplanted from *other* relationships. My patients have responded emotionally to me as they would to a father, brother or lover. Interpreting the dramas taking place between us allows them to better understand their lives.

Terminating, as distressing as it can be, also yields rich understandings. The end of a therapy can cause a patient's deeply rooted feelings about commitment, separation and even death to surface. Exploring these can help patients deal with the fact that human relationships change, and sometimes end.

The process of saying goodbye allowed the first patient to further confront the fear she experienced when her husband passed away. "As long as my husband was living," she said during one of our last sessions, "I wasn't afraid of anything. When he got sick, my source of strength vanished. Your leaving makes me feel that way, again."

"But you were able to care for your husband when he became ill," I said. "You survived losing him. And you've come to terms with your children leaving home."

"Well," she said, "What choice did I have?"

"Someone else might have given up. You didn't. I think you've been drawing on an inner strength most of your life."

She nodded slowly. "I guess my brother didn't manage to beat everything out of me."

"That inner strength didn't die with your husband, either. And it won't end with this therapy."

"It sometimes feels that way, though," she said. She smiled. "I guess I'll always find a way to keep going."

Later I wondered: "What would keep me going?" In the weeks preceding my last clinic day, I battled extreme feelings of guilt and sadness. The connections I had made with patients had sustained me, too. As I struggled to help them examine their feelings about my leaving, I had to deal with my own feelings as well.

I wondered whether part of the intensity of these reactions was transplanted from my personal life. Why was it, for instance, that some of the patients I found it hardest to terminate with were women in their sixties—the same age as my mother?

One of my supervisors, particularly sensitive to the difficulties with goodbyes in psychiatric practice, was especially supportive. "This once," he said, "finish something cleanly. You owe it to yourself. Don't nickel and dime this transition. Move on."

Interestingly, I got the most help from a young man I had been treating for paranoid schizophrenia. He had remained nearly silent during many of our meetings but was visibly moved as our last hour ended. "I'll miss seeing you," he said, extending his hand. "Be careful."

I shook his hand. "I'll be careful," I said. "I'll miss you, too."

He turned around as he was leaving the office and stood in the doorway. "I'm not going to believe those damn voices, anymore," he said. "I'm not going to listen to them. I'll be all right . . . if you will."

"That's a deal," I said.

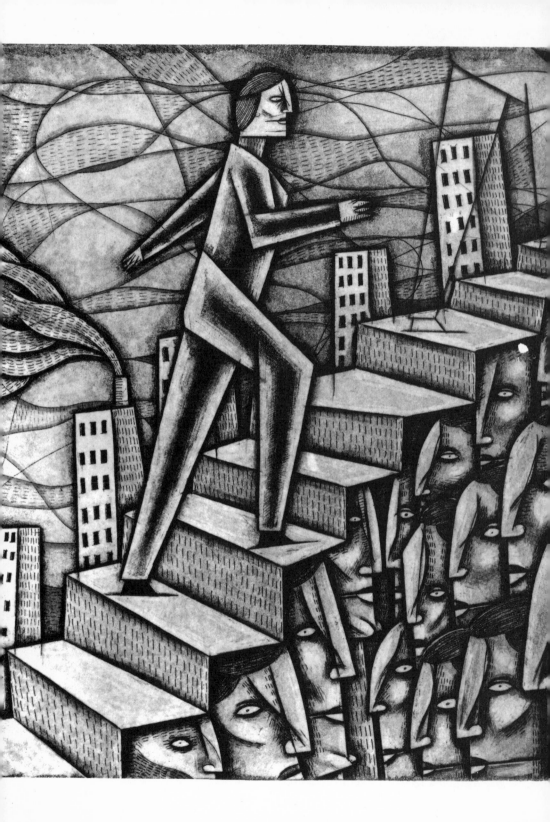

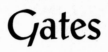Gates

13

The Gatekeeper

Believe me, if you mean the trouble, if you mean people with money and others without and people with time and others without and others with good liquor and others without and others with fine places to sleep and others without, believe me I don't understand it. If you mean, even, one man and one woman, together, married or not married or in love or not in love, let me apologize. If I've given the impression that I'm one who knows or one who would be apt to know, I didn't mean to. I don't know. I can't make head or tail of it.

William Saroyan   "For My Part I'll Smoke
a Good Ten Cent Cigar"

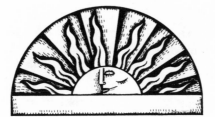

Shortly after 1 A.M. recently, on call in the psychiatric emergency room of a Boston hospital, I was asked to evaluate a homeless man and, in the process, confronted the limits of my professional empathy.

My beeper had woken me after 20 minutes of sleep, and the emergency room nurse at the Boston Veterans Administration Hospital handed me a consultation form on which she had written the identifying information: 56-year-old, divorced, homeless veteran complaining of depression; history of alcohol dependence, no apparent suicidal or homicidal impulses.

The negatives surprised me a bit. Many homeless veterans who know the VA hospital system and need a place to sleep have learned to claim emphatically that they are feeling suicidal or homicidal. Hospital beds are at such a premium that any psychiatric problem short of life and death usually is made to wait until normal business hours.

Against a constant flow of would-be inpatients, one of my roles as a resident physician is that of gatekeeper, evaluating the veracity of suicidal or homicidal threats, attempting to defuse empty threats in order to justify keeping the ward census at a reasonable number.

After nights when I have not admitted any patients, I have been congratulated by colleagues, slapped on the back and affectionately called a "wall."

But this man was a newcomer to the emergency room; he didn't know how to manipulate the system. He had only recently lost his job, then his wife, then his home. For a month he had wandered, drinking to forget, sleeping in shelters. But tonight he had sobered up too late to secure a shelter bed, and, alone in the freezing wind, he felt his grief and exhaustion weighing more heavily than ever.

"I need to be in the hospital," he told me. "I have to get a handle on myself."

I listened at length to his description of the losses he had suffered. "Have things gotten so bad for you that you've thought of hurting yourself?" I asked.

"I would never do that," he replied.

"Some people get so angry that they start thinking of hurting someone else."

"Look, doc, I'm worn out. Period. I'm not mad at anyone but myself."

He denied symptoms of clinical depression or any other major mental illness. His intellect and memory were normal. He had never been admitted to a psychiatric hospital and took no medication for emotional problems. As if to offer something to reward my search for symptoms, he showed me his feet, skinned and bloody from walking the streets.

"There's no question you need help with the problems you've talked about," I said. "I can help you follow up with the outpatient clinic downtown."

He took the slip of paper on which I had written the clinic's address and phone number. "I don't need to be in the hospital?" he asked, plaintively.

"No," I said. "But I'd like to be sure you'll make an appointment with the clinic. They may decide to schedule an admission in the future."

"I will," he nodded. He looked at me expectantly. "Where do I go now?"

Sometimes the answer to that question is simple, but not this time. None of the shelters the night hospital staff called had any beds available. The admitting office of the hospital had no room to house another patient on a ward. The security guard reluctantly reminded me that no one was allowed to sleep overnight in the hospital lobby. The buses to the airport, where homeless people have told me they sometimes find safe corners, had stopped running. The hospital's petty cash fund had run dry.

"I can't find a place anywhere for you," I said, after nearly an hour, shaking my head.

"It's cold," he said. "It'll be four, five hours before it's light."

I reached into the pocket of my scrubs and handed him three dollar bills. "Maybe the subway?" I suggested.

He started putting his socks over the medicated gauze I had wrapped around his injured feet. "The subway's dangerous," he said.

I stood up. "I wouldn't want to be there myself, but there's not a lot more I can do."

That was a lie, of course, and I believe we both knew it. I'd only part with three dollars for a person in no immediate danger with nowhere to go.

The two twenties upstairs in my call room—enough for a taxi and a motel—stayed there. My car, good shelter from the wind, was parked right out front. I didn't even think of unlocking it for him. I have family and friends who live not 30 minutes from the hospital, with extra beds. I wouldn't think of asking them to open their homes to a stranger. And as a psychiatrist, empathy is my calling.

Why wouldn't I do more? The reason is that I had hit my internal "wall." Part of it was fear. I have learned that I really don't know much about anyone after an hour.

Moreover, despite all my attempts to banish it, I still harbor the prejudice that those who cannot sustain themselves in society are less likely to be bound by society's rules. Losing all one's possessions raises the suspicion that a person is somehow out of control in every way.

I felt—unfairly or not—that to get involved with this patient would put me at risk of being physically harmed or at least exploited. Maybe I was afraid of being overwhelmed, that if I truly extended myself to one homeless man, what would prevent my being used up by the sheer bulk of homeless people?

As a child, I was more than once admonished by a teacher not to share candy with a friend if I didn't have enough for everyone. So I kept it to myself.

I believe I also had myself convinced that my restraint had a therapeutic component. Perhaps, I thought, this man had not yet fallen far enough to take hold of himself, to stop drinking, to get another job. And even if he didn't spend the money on booze, a room tonight might be no more than a bandage obscuring an infected sore, allowing whatever infection was at work to do more lasting damage. What, indeed, if his disorder was a dependent personality? I would be playing into his pathological inability to be self-sufficient.

The problem is that these are theories.

I know there are many people who need to be taken care of. But at 2 A.M. the job of distinguishing those who need firm limits from those who need warm beds from those who need to be left alone is overwhelming.

So I am left with the nagging guilt that I could, or should, have done more for this man.

14

Sex in Psychotherapy

I found myself in a dark wood,
For I had lost the right path.

Dante Alighieri   *Inferno*

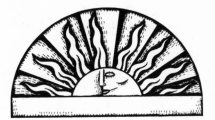

*I*t is conceivable that at some point in my career I will want to have a sexual relationship with a patient. I don't believe that such a relationship could be therapeutic for the woman, nor do I imagine it could be the prelude to lasting love.

I agree it could do irreparable harm to both patient and therapist. I know that this kind of behavior is specifically proscribed by the American Psychiatric Association and the Massachusetts Board of Registration in Medicine. I agree that it is professionally unethical. It also violates my personal ethics.

In treating dozens of patients over the past three years, I have felt physically attracted to only one. During weekly psychotherapy sessions, she began wearing revealing clothing and hinting that we could meet outside the office. While I understood her behavior as a compulsion to replay an episode of childhood sexual abuse by her father, it took perseverance for me to repeatedly interpret it, rather than to let it pass without comment.

My success in helping her to understand her provocative behavior rather than participating in it with her, however, does not predict with absolute certainty that I will always react professionally. Barbara Forsch, now a psychotherapist herself, has described in a book an interaction she had with her own therapist years earlier that ended in a sexual relationship:

> I went to my third session . . . with my raincoat on and nothing but underwear underneath. When it was time to go, I took my coat off and rubbed up against him. He was kind of passive about it, but I could tell that he was going to let it keep happening. It just escalated from there. But now I see that everything that pushed me to be sexual with him was with me before I ever walked into his office . . .
>
> He could have said he wasn't going to have sex with me. He could have said, "I see what you're doing, and I totally understand, but I can't do this with you. Let's talk about what goes on inside you that you have to do this."

I'd like to think that I wouldn't make the same mistake her therapist did, but I can't predict exactly how I would react. Nor is my profession's track record particularly comforting. Therapist-patient sex is common. Studies show that as many as 5 to 10 percent of my colleagues—the vast majority of them men—have transgressed. One study by psychiatrist Nannette Gartrell found that more than 16 percent of these liaisons continued longer than five years. Sixty-five percent of the psychiatrists stated that they had fallen in love with the patients with whom they became involved.

There are, clearly, malevolent psychiatrists, psychologists, social workers and clergy who knowingly abuse their power. I am more interested in those who, despite good intentions, nonetheless harm their patients. I empathize with them because I know we are human and our work places us at the breaking point of powerful and sometimes unpredictable emotional tides.

One risk I have already identified is that the level of understanding at which I arrive with patients is in many cases deeper than that which I achieve with friends or even family members. Discovering with patients their true hopes and fears makes me feel close to them. I can understand how such intimacy with a woman, which since boyhood I have associated with romance, can lead to physical contact.

Moreover, there are irrational attachments that lie in wait. My patients and I come to therapy with feelings about others—parents or children or lovers—that are routinely displaced onto the therapeutic relationship. A woman may, for example, have feelings for her therapist that actually originate in her relationship with her father. Conversely, a therapist may react to a patient with emotions stemming from a long-past romance.

Indeed, these displaced feelings are generally regarded as so powerful that a patient is presumed incapable by the legal system of granting informed consent for a sexual relationship. That is why therapists who have sex with patients who later sue them are often found guilty of malpractice and why a growing number of states are criminalizing such behavior.

Identifying these phenomena and interpreting them is, of course, the therapist's stock-in-trade. Still, I doubt that even long experience with these intense emotional forces makes us uniformly invulnerable to them.

I have the benefits of good health, close friends and a loving family. But I imagine that terrible losses in my life could weaken me and make it more appealing to reach out inappropriately.

Peter Rutter, a San Francisco psychiatrist, writes in his book *Sex in the Forbidden Zone* about his own difficulty refusing the advances of a young, beautiful woman he was treating.

While crying over the humiliation of having recently been rejected by a man, she left her chair and moved toward his own. She brushed against him and rested her head on his lap:

> My likelihood of collaborating in this sexual scenario was enhanced by the fact that, because of losses in my own personal life, I had been feeling quite depressed that winter, and I had no place to go that evening except back to the empty house where I live alone . . .
> I knew that by doing nothing at all, I could simply allow Mia to touch me in what was certainly going to be a sexual way. I could passively accede to her agenda, letting my depression mirror her own, allowing us to become wounded patients together."

Rutter directed the patient back to her seat, but not before struggling silently with his desires.

It would be simpler for society to respond to transgression by therapists if those who engaged in sexual relationships with patients were evil manipulators, rather than inept or vulnerable. Then the only task would be to mete out punishment. And it seems to me that society is embracing that easy answer.

Several states, including California, Colorado, Maine, Minnesota, North Dakota, and Wisconsin, now have statutes making therapist-patient sex a felony, rather than malpractice.

Public outrage seems to greet nearly every publicized case. The obvious presumption is that the psychiatrist, trusted to act in the best interest of the patient, has taken advantage of his or her power. After coaxing the woman (usually) to reveal her true self, he has manipulated her into fulfilling his own base needs.

There is no question that therapist-patient sex is bad medicine. One study reported that a majority of psychiatrists who had been physically intimate with their own therapists thought of the experience as harmful.

In another study, 90 percent of patients who had engaged in sexual relations with a previous therapist were assessed by their current therapist as having suffered negative effects. These may include flashbacks, nightmares, inability to trust and increased risk of suicide.

The problem is that labeling all the doctors involved as depraved or criminal may oversimplify the problem. It may be that the emotions raised in therapy can derail even skilled psychiatrists of normally high character.

Understanding this would not excuse an offending psychiatrist's behavior, but it might make clearer the enormity of the task of predicting and preventing it.

15

One of the Boys

The great question . . . which I have not been able to answer, despite my thirty years of research into the feminine soul, is "What does a woman want?"

Sigmund Freud

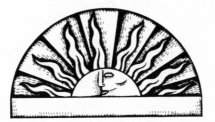

The smoke around the confirmation of Clarence Thomas as Supreme Court Justice may have cleared, but the volcano grumbling beneath all the captivating sparks is still active. Whatever happened or did not happen to Professor Anita Hill, the narrow focus of the hearings on blatant sexual harassment belies the smoldering resentment and aggression deeply felt by a large percentage of men toward the accomplished women with whom they interact.

Nearly all the environments in which I have worked or studied, from college and medical school classrooms to hospitals to media corporations, have included a masculine subculture—well educated and genteel—that encourages views of women as sexually needy or confused, emotionally unbalanced and potentially self-destructive.

This masculine subculture has several related tenets. First, it holds that career motivation in a woman who does not temper her ambition with flirtation represents an abnormal displacement of sexual desire into occupational advancement. Second, it makes the case, often as a what-she-needs jest, that a woman's intellectual and professional energy can be quelled by providing her with good-enough sex. Third, it casts women as the unfortunate victims of unwieldy hormones likely responsible for displays of anger or stereotypically male toughness.

For men, membership in the club is frequently offered by senior staff members. They make clear, through their own off-color remarks, that the sexist posture of junior colleagues will place them in no real peril and may, in fact, make them one of the inner circle.

At a business meeting I attended, for example, a female colleague was the sole critic of a proposal being presented. After some debate, during which she became rather caustic, the meeting adjourned.

Several of us were left, gathering our papers. "One of you guys needs to help her out after hours," a supervisor of mine chuckled. "She's wound up."

No man these days is a naive recipient of such an overture. Part of the reason is that sexism is endemic in our culture. We are educated in a society that cultivates a passive, rather than equal, role for women. It dictates, for example, that females should adorn themselves with makeup and earrings, remove body hair and eschew contact sports. Racks of magazines displaying naked women greet boys in variety stores.

Clichés about women are not just sexual but psychological. A pervasive social stereotype has long existed of women as masochistic, propelled toward abuse by a psychological connection to the pain of childbirth, a vulnerable anatomy and an inevitable internal conflict between the desire to reproduce and the desire to remain chaste and apart from men.

A 1970s edition, for example, of the textbook *Obstetrics and Gynecology* stated that "every aspect of a woman's life is colored" by this "ability to accept the masochism that is part of her feminine role." In a later edition, this passage was deleted, but the outmoded stereotype persists.

Women sometimes declare themselves "free" of these conflicts by claiming an uneasy associate membership in the male subculture. They do so by making their own sexually derogatory remarks about themselves or other women. This lends an unfortunate air of credibility to the subculture's prejudices.

In the dozens of back-room men's club gatherings to which I have been privy, no one has ever fully broken ranks with the group by strenuously objecting to the degradation of a woman.

The lack of vocal opposition is multifaceted. To many men, sexist remarks can read like tests of faith, in that refusing the implied camaraderie will lead others to doubt their sexual prowess. Participating in this reduction of women to objects is offered as proof of manliness.

Some theorists would say that unresolved feelings about homosexuality are raised when men work together. Sexist jokes serve to fuel graphic confirmations of heterosexuality.

Perhaps more powerful and insidious, however, is that basking in the subculture can feel warm and familiar. It not only creates a host of allies but also recalls unrestrained boyhood locker-room talk and the high school postulate that winning a girl's affection is never worth losing a buddy.

It took a great deal of introspection for me to recognize, then partly understand, the paradoxical warmth and distaste I used to feel when hearing sexist remarks. I remember the teasing I endured from grade school bullies, who were quick to detect my school phobia (a fear of school, often reflecting an ambivalence about separating from parents). This early isolation from my peers has predisposed me to revel in acceptance as *one of the boys*.

Some psychoanalysts would say that the need of some men to diminish females, particularly female authority figures, lies even deeper, in remnants of anger about the level of control exercised by their mothers. There may also be lingering frustration over maintaining intimacy without sexually consummating the mother-son relationship. It should come as no surprise, viewed through the lens of these theories, that offhand sexual comments about powerful women can provoke giggling from 50-year-old men.

Another reservoir of male anger may be the traditional female role in screening potential sexual partners. The proper right of women to accept or refuse advances makes them instant authority figures. Women can say no. This might partly explain the frequency with which men half-joke about female authority figures that "she needs to be bent over the desk."

What seems clear is that these conscious and unconscious issues are pervasive and largely ignored. We know too little about the dynamics of sexism directed against women.

Dramatic hearings and stringent rules of decorum may change the landscape of male-female interactions, but, until we commit ourselves to full study of the underlying emotional conflicts, they will continue to smolder underground.

16

Fatal Afflictions

He casually raised his open hand and tapped the knife a little deeper. After he put another little bit of the blade in his chest, he almost smiled. . . . He leaned just perceptibly. "You don't have to worry about this. I don't want you to worry about this." . . .

"Why?" I said.

"The knife feels good."

. . . He said something else, but I didn't hear him. I knew it was hopeless. I could not have said it then, but I knew in my bones that he was caught in a life where the only thing left to do was what he was doing. He had told himself a story he believed, or somebody else had told it to him, a story in which the next thing that happened—the only thing that *could* happen—was the knife.

Harry Crews *A Childhood: The Biography of a Place*

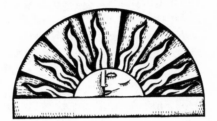

Recently, I attended my first postmortem for a psychiatric patient. The goal of a postmortem is to gather and review the course of a patient's fatal illness. As a medical student, I attended several for patients who died of cancer, AIDS or heart disease and learned that, even after medicine's most heroic efforts, death sometimes prevails.

This postmortem lacked that degree of peace with death. Despite the efforts of many who had helped the patient survive decades of severe mental illness, punctuated by repeated suicide attempts, there was little of the resignation I remember sharing with internists and surgeons who spoke of having done the best they could.

The reality that seems too hard for psychiatrists to accept is that the best drugs we have, all the empathy we muster and the social supports we erect will not be enough to keep some patients alive.

More than in many other specialties, a treatment failure in psychiatry can feel like a personal defeat for the therapist. Although psychiatry is based on the medical model—that certain symptoms comprise syndromes that call for specific treatments—few psychiatrists believe that what we do can be described—or prescribed—in cookbook form. A cardiologist, for example, can be reassured that he or she prescribed the proper drugs prior to a patient's tragic heart attack. It happened anyhow.

By contrast, psychiatrists are trained to know the power of emotional connections, the poetry of interpersonal relations. What we do is arguably as much art as science. Many of us may never be able to convince ourselves that we did everything that could be done for a patient who commits suicide. There are always those nagging doubts: Did we miss an important theme in the therapy? Were we too wedded to professionalism when the patient needed reassurance and love?

Many of us worry that perhaps someone else could have kept the patient alive. The isolation in which we work magnifies the natural doubts many of us have about our abilities. It seems harder for psychiatrists than specialists in other fields to assess accurately their proficiency. Medical and surgical residents generally agree on who among them is most skilled.

Psychiatry residents can't do much more than guess. Our work goes on behind closed doors, sometimes for years. The goals are individual. Success or failure is not easily measured.

One of the patients I treated earlier in my training killed himself while still in the hospital. As is routine in residency, I had rotated to another service several months prior to his suicide, and his care had become the responsibility of another resident. Even so, I still wondered whether I could have done something to prevent his death.

I had not visited him since my transfer from that hospital. Maybe I should have. Perhaps I should have made it plain that, upon his discharge, I would see him as an outpatient, but I didn't.

This patient had suffered terribly for decades. After his illness began, he couldn't work. He found it extremely difficult to form or sustain any relationship. He felt completely empty and alone and spent most of his time in the hospital.

Sometimes I think he's better off now, although some of my colleagues might regard my saying so as heretical, a premature and unwarranted admission of defeat.

Physicians find it easier to see relief in death when the pain is physical and the organism is visibly decaying. We are much more reluctant to acknowledge that emotional pain and loss of life spirit can become unbearable.

The most obvious reason is that few of us have a clear idea how it feels to suffer with illnesses like schizophrenia or major depression. I have heard psychosis described as being a passenger on a plane perpetually about to crash, but I can't quite imagine it.

Accepting that emotional pain can become intolerable means risking a precedent. How much pain would be considered sufficient justification for suicide?

From the beginning of our training, doctors are instilled with the belief that death is the enemy and must be vanquished. Acknowledging that this might not always be the right thing to do means unleashing a confusing welter of ethical and emotional questions.

Another emotion in the aftermath of a patient's suicide is anger, not unlike that experienced by friends and relatives. How could we not feel unappreciated, abandoned, inadequate and embarrassed in front of our peers?

In many instances, suicide doesn't seem to be a rational response to a hopeless situation but is a clear symptom of mental illness. Depression, for example, can create feelings that one is evil and deserves to die. Schizophrenia can cause voices that command patients to kill themselves. When the thoughts or voices are silenced by psychotherapy and medicine, the person's genuine and strong will to live is often revealed.

A highly decorated World War II veteran was admitted to my service with a psychotic depression. He was often tearful, had no appetite and couldn't sleep. Although he had an unusually distinguished military record, he decided he was a coward. Honor, he felt, dictated that he kill himself. His suicidal thoughts were clearly a symptom of his illness.

From him and others I have learned not to rely exclusively on psychotherapy to reach patients during such acute episodes of major mental illness. The individual's ability to relate to his or her therapist and to benefit from connecting the past with the present is too often impaired. As clinicians, we use some of the distance that treating the brain with drugs allows.

But that distance can close unpredictably. A patient might recover, only to fall prey to recurrent depression. The episodes, despite treatment, might become darker, longer and more frequent. The person underneath that illness, a person I may have come to know intimately, could reach out and touch me with his unbearable suffering.

Psychiatrists respond to that touch, which may be the greatest reason we cannot achieve professional distance from a patient's death. The work itself ensnares us. With all the attention to maintaining the structure of the therapeutic relationship, all the emphasis on the symbolic importance of money changing hands, all the limits on disclosing our personal lives, we sometimes grow to love our patients.

We may pick a technical term for that emotion or try to explain it away as part of the dynamics of treatment. But when a postmortem feels a little like a funeral, the difference seems a matter of semantics.

17

Souled: Money and Therapy

Certainly there are lots of things in life that money won't buy, but it's very funny—Have you ever tried to buy them without money?

Ogden Nash "Happy Days"

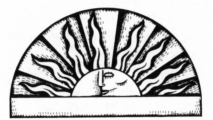

One of my patients recently informed me that she had decided to charge for sex. After many affairs with men who had proven untrustworthy, she was abandoning her search for a genuine relationship.

"If you're all rats," she explained, "I might as well get some money for my time."

A week before, we had spoken about whether she would be able to afford care at the clinic when her insurance coverage ran out. She made it clear that she would discontinue treatment if she had to pay a single dollar out-of-pocket.

I felt the two issues were connected. "Do you think your decision to sell yourself is related to the thought of paying to see me?" I asked.

"I'd just be selling my body," she said, smiling.

I rent my soul. Patients who have the money must pay for me to listen to them and to help them make sense of their lives. Even when the feelings between us mimic parenthood or friendship, even if they truly border on love, patients must continue to pay or our relationship will come to an end.

My father, who has spent his life in sales, once challenged me to understand the difference between a calling and a job. "You, God willing, won't have to sell anything," I remember him saying to me.

I chose medicine partly for the luxury of earning a living by serving a basic human need rather than competing to create an artificial one. But I am finding traffic in empathy especially troubling.

My conscience should be calmed by tradition. Freud, who was ostracized by Viennese physicians for refusing charity cases, believed that his patients could not be helped unless they paid a fair price for treatment. The exchange of money defined the interaction as both professional and valuable.

Money continues to be regarded as a critical part of the therapeutic process. It helps to prevent the relationship from wandering toward friendship, violating the distance required for dispassionate observation. As part of this rigid structure, the issue of payment can even illuminate other conflicts in a patient's life. The therapist may, for example, be imbued with attributes of a withholding parent. Issues of social power and position may be unearthed and discussed.

Indeed, some psychiatrists believe that dispensing free care would shift the balance of power precariously in the therapist's direction, holding us out as secular saints somehow above the fray.

Knowing all this, and even enjoying the distance of a salaried trainee, I still feel embarrassed when my patients mention clinic fees. No matter how much I care for a patient, the fact that dollars are the life blood of the relationship seems to color my concern as impure—a hint of the prostitute feigning romance. My heart tells me it is wrong to charge to help someone who, having shared intimate details of his or her life, has become part of mine.

Moreover, I have not noticed that the state hospital patients I serve, who pay no fee, benefit from my services any less. Nor has any scientific study proven that paying for treatment has any therapeutic value.

A middle-aged woman I treated lost her job after meeting with me weekly for many months. She had not paid for several visits. When the secretary reminded her of her balance, she stormed out of the clinic and never returned.

I might have regarded the rage my patient felt at the mention of her bill as an irrational association of me with her cold and insensitive father. My professional distance had become an intolerable symbol of love denied. Money had served a purpose by becoming the screen upon which she had projected a real conflict.

But it seemed equally possible that our relationship had evolved to a point at which the exchange of money was, in fact, a kind of love denied. I knew her well and cared about her. We were connected. For a price. Therapy seemed more like another trauma than a repetition of a previous betrayal.

I have wondered whether any of my discomfort about money lies in my own doubt about the value of the services I provide. An ophthalmologist can restore vision by removing cataracts. The gain is immediate and objective. The benefits of my services are subjective. Patients may or may not find months of treatment helpful. My skills sometimes result in rapid and dramatic resolution of symptoms like psychosis, but more often they result in slow, subtle change. Sometimes I am unsure whether we have made any progress at all.

I don't believe that these feelings are the core of my concern. The intrusion of commerce bothers me most, in fact, when the usefulness of therapy is apparent, and the connection between myself and a patient is strong. I feel worst charging for the best hour. My worry is not whether our work together is effective enough to merit payment, but whether it is too deeply moving to charge for.

I wouldn't have nearly the trouble handing someone a pill and billing for it. Medicine is a tangible product; dispensing it introduces an accepted commercial entity—the pharmaceutical company—into the exchange. But demanding money for understanding, which is mine to dispense as I choose, makes me feel that I am withholding the help that any good person would offer another in pain.

As a boy, I resented my temple charging for seats to services at Yom Kippur and Rosh Hashanah. Even though the poor were admitted free of charge, I didn't think anyone should pay to participate in something spiritual. The connection between my feelings about money, religion and psychiatry is not mere coincidence. It is the spiritual aspect of psychotherapy that I wish to insulate from commerce.

I think my protective feelings are justified. Psychiatry is falling in line with government and insurance company reimbursement policies based on the medical model of targeted, time-limited treatments aimed at specific syndromes. Pharmaceutical companies are funding massive research projects demonstrating the efficacy of psychiatric drugs. The examined life turns out to be hard to defend as cost-effective. So psychiatry's perspective, in what we choose to learn and to teach, is shifting.

We don't record grief as an admitting diagnosis anymore. We must find a similar condition in a psychiatric catalogue of five-digit codes and enter the corresponding number. Otherwise, the insurance company won't pay.

So how can psychiatry respond?

We can refuse the language of science when it fails to describe what we do. We can argue that mental health means more than the absence of catalogued diseases, that insight is at once valuable and hard to quantify by cost. We can learn a lesson about the limits of trade in human interactions. We can push for increased and equal access to psychiatric care for all.

Psychiatry's wink at economics, the peace we have made marrying empathy and money, may ultimately erode the moral and spiritual underpinnings of the field. We defended payment as a necessary component of the therapeutic relationship, insisting it reflected the real world and could enhance our objectivity. But I believe it was always at odds with the heart of our work. If we had examined the conflict more deeply, we could have avoided some of the losses we have suffered as a result.

18

Ministering to the Spirit

Beyond all question there are persons in whom . . . the higher condition, having reached the due degree of energy, bursts through all barriers and sweeps in like a sudden flood. These are the most striking and memorable cases, the cases of instantaneous conversion to which the conception of divine grace has been most peculiarly attached.

William James   *The Varieties of Religious Experience*

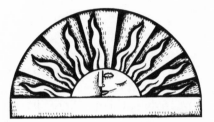

Some time during the second year of my training in psychiatry, I began to understand how my patients' early life experiences, long forgotten and unearthed only through psychotherapy, were continuing to influence their lives. I became suddenly and unshakably attached to the belief that powerful, unconscious mental processes connected me with their suffering. The knowledge became greater than the sum of its parts; I was warmed by a new confidence that man has a soul and that we are related, one to another, by an emotional existence that may survive even death.

I can sometimes sense the new calm in junior residents when this knowledge gently touches, then embraces them. We speak to one another of finally understanding what our work is all about.

Having undergone this personal evolution in the name of science and medicine, I now understand why Sigmund Freud would have raged, as he did, against what he called the illusions underlying religion. Psychoanalytic thought and religious faith have been, from the beginning, close cousins, competing for the same spiritual ground.

Freud believed religious stories were fairy tales, which devotees irrationally treated "as if" they were fact. He believed these "as if" myths would ultimately be rejected because they could not be authenticated. "They give the name 'God,'" Freud complained, "to some vague abstraction, which they have created for themselves."

But Freud himself created "as if" truths. He hypothesized the organization of the human psyche into what he called ego (negotiator), id (instinctive drive) and superego (social and moral values). The ego acted as a kind of mediator between, for example, the sex drive of the id and moral commitments of the superego. Imbalances among the three led to certain forms of psychological pain.

This organization, however, cannot be proved scientifically. None of these components of the mind can be visualized, weighed or touched. They constitute a powerful and useful parable that seems to explain elements of human distress. As such, they are not wholly different from biblical stories that also describe the struggle between good and evil in man. They feel like truth to those who believe.

The notion of an all-powerful God, Freud asserted, springs from man's desire to understand and feel secure amidst the chaos of nature and fate. Again, psychoanalytic theory offered its own brand of security in the form of psychic determinism: the theory that, through guided introspection, seemingly random life events could be shown to have unstated meaning and purpose, often linked to the past. While these links in time are intuitively appealing, they cannot ultimately be proven or refuted.

Transference, the process by which patients unconsciously invest their therapists with qualities that actually belong to important figures from childhood, provides similar insulation from the fact that love and life are fleeting. Through transference, human connections, like emotional viruses, can survive indefinitely and incorporate themselves in entirely new relationships.

Dreams, too, are demystified by relating them to emotionally charged issues from wakefulness. In this way, sleep, so often connected symbolically with death, is tied securely to conscious life.

To me, and to many psychiatrists, such ideas do seem like fact because they are such powerful tools of understanding and healing. Indeed, those who reject the influence of early life experience on adult decisions and dismiss the power of unconscious mental processes sometimes strike us as psychological heathens, blind to higher truths. If they would simply "let it happen," they would be released from the bondage of their concrete thinking.

Is it any wonder, then, that medical students considering careers in psychiatry often struggle with the feeling that they are, at once, stepping toward and away from science? Some actually worry how to break the news to parents. They sense that, far from simply choosing the brain as their organ of special interest, they are choosing a different mode of thinking and, perhaps, a way of life.

Even the mental state associated with performing and receiving psychotherapy has elements in common with that achieved by some people through prayer. Moments when I feel an intense emotional connection with patients, precisely because they seem inexplicable through science, fill me with wonder and a sense of inner peace.

Our mode of listening is, in some ways, ministerial. We are convinced of the emotional dynamics at work in life and unflappably wait and watch for these to become manifest to patients. An obviously meaningful slip of the tongue, for example, can seem to fill the room with awesome evidence of the unconscious. Again and again, patients of mine reflect that our meetings remind them of church confession. Details like the quiet of the clinic and the persistence of incandescent lighting (when fluorescent lighting dominates elsewhere in the hospital) do nothing to weaken the comparison.

Psychiatry's fierce commitment to confidentiality, the prohibition of therapist-patient sexual contact and my own discomfort with the exchange of money for therapy further suggest to me that I work at once in the house of medicine and the house of God.

That this spiritual foundation coexists with advances in neuropharmacology and brain imaging techniques and genetics is the source of much of the excitement and much of the angst in psychiatry. While the field as a whole is becoming increasingly technical, the theories Freud developed turn out to have a life completely independent of science. The notion that they would ultimately yield smoothly to a scientific understanding of the brain was clearly flawed.

We remain infinitely far from biological explanations of how the mind can relegate early trauma to the unconscious, how such experiences can continue to shape our lives and how words can heal.

The question now is how psychiatry as a medical specialty can remain hospitable enough to spiritual thinking. The tension between mind cures and brain cures is real. Forces outside the profession, such as cutbacks in insurance reimbursement, are making it increasingly difficult to offer insight-oriented psychotherapy in the medical environment. And psychiatry's own rush to get in step with such financial imperatives favors quicker, relatively less expensive, easily documented forms of treatment.

If the tension becomes too great, those convinced of the power of Freud's ideas might, like refugees from other forms of intolerance, find themselves searching for another home beyond the shores of medicine. The foundation for a kind of therapeutic, cognitive clergy is, after all, already built.

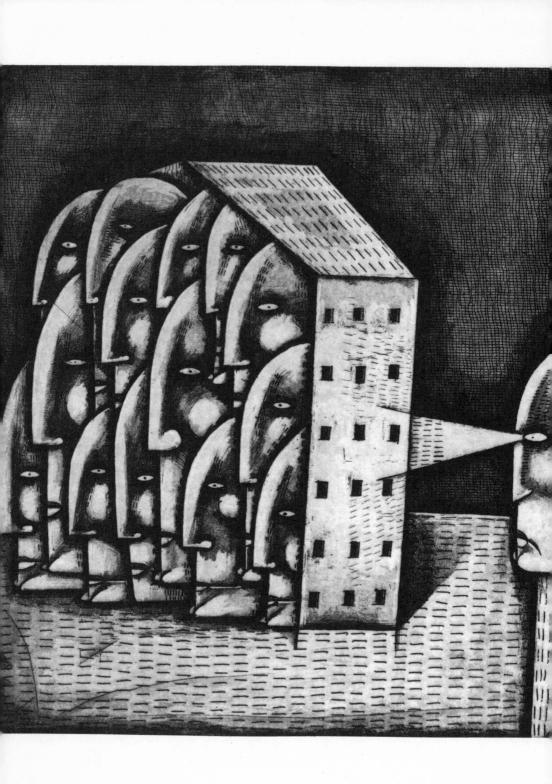

My Brother's Keeper

19

My Brother's Keeper: The Dilemmas of Medical Guardianship

Am I my brother's keeper?

The Old Testament

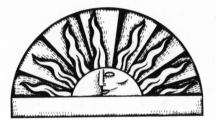

The most frightening part of helping to take away a psychiatric patient's right to make decisions is that I'm getting good at it.

I have learned how to formulate a patient's history and recount the details of his or her present illness and worrisome behavior in a way that makes the risks of free choice—of liberty—unacceptable to a judge. I make the court comfortable with the notion of the state as parent. There are key facts I highlight—a history of assault or self-destructiveness or caution thrown dangerously and unpredictably to the winds.

I am new at this, a senior resident in psychiatry, yet I have never been denied.

The patients for whom psychiatrists seek medical guardians are generally those at risk of harm, who either refuse widely accepted treatments or are too disorganized or sick to reliably see them through.

We must be convinced that mental illness has so disrupted the patient's thought processes that he or she cannot rationally elect or reject the alternatives we present. Sometimes, the guardianship is temporary—just long enough to get through a period of worsening symptoms. When the likelihood of restoring the patient's safety and reliability is remote, however, guardianship can be permanent.

I agonize abut removing my preconceptions from the process, trying to make sure that I'm not making judgments about what is appropriate, only about what is dangerous. But I am never completely at peace taking such action. From boyhood, my personal evolution has been an ever-increasing bias for the individual and against the status quo. I strongly empathize with people who cannot comply with the demands of society, believing as I do that society itself is deeply flawed and insensitive. No wonder that I bristle at the gates between what we label eccentric, what we call sick and what we brand, finally, as incompetent.

The legal environment is foreign to me. I feel out of place in a courtroom, designed as it is for defense and prosecution. I dislike watching my patient listening to my testimony, as if we were opponents, when the truth is that my gut sinks when I think the lawyers' questions might hurt my patient's feelings. What I love about psychiatry is building alliances and trust. What could be a more graphic representation of my failure than a courtroom?

Some cases are easier than others. One of the easiest concerned a schizophrenic and diabetic patient who had repeatedly stopped taking his antipsychotic medication. He was a big, brawling man and he felt the medicine weakened him physically. It probably did. Unfortunately, when he stopped taking the antipsychotic drug, he began to feel indestructible and also refused to take his insulin. He was transferred to my ward from the intensive care unit, where he had received emergency treatment for ketoacidosis, a sometimes fatal complication of uncontrolled diabetes.

The clarity of the danger against the cloudiness of my patient's insight made illness my clear opponent. I was fighting to preserve a vulnerable person against a faceless intruder that had nearly taken his life. Two against one; we were a team, even if he couldn't quite see it that way. I read his unwillingness to accept a guardian voluntarily as inability to acknowledge weakness, to come to terms with the constraints of his illness. And I told him so.

The judge listened to my testimony and heard the danger. He ordered a temporary guardian who would monitor the patient's medications and consent, in his place, to medical and psychiatric treatment. The guardianship would be reevaluated after 60 days. I felt I had performed a good service. All the more when my patient thanked me and shook my hand.

The art of inviting the courts into psychiatric treatment is in preserving a relationship with the patient, despite the adversarial nature of the process.

It isn't always easy for me to choose sides. The hardest cases are those in which the danger is more remote, and I question how much psychiatry can truly offer the patient in exchange for dependence.

What if the medicines work poorly or inflict severe side effects? What if the patient's life, albeit colored by the limitations and dangers that attend mental illness, is nonetheless more full than it would be once legally bound to the system?

In such cases, I am relieved that decisions to pursue guardianship are made by a treatment team, including senior physicians, and that the judge—not the medical expert—is the final arbiter. I take an emotional step back.

I cared for an elderly man who suffered from mania, a disorder of mood marked by too much energy, a disturbing rush of ideas and, often, grossly impaired judgment. He read voraciously, traveled state to state and especially enjoyed discussing, at lightning speed, current events. Unfortunately, he also trespassed frequently and approached random strangers as friends. Rejecting the notion that he was ill, he refused all medications and energetically argued that he should be allowed to leave the hospital.

Reigning this patient in hurt me because I found his intellect lively and his naiveté charming. I was moved by his protest for freedom. It took guidance from the treatment team to help me balance the benefits of maintaining his free choice against the risks of his innocence in an unfriendly world. They helped me to see the pain behind his seemingly carefree demeanor and to see his illness as the real impediment. We proceeded successfully toward treatment. But I felt uneasy all along the way.

Sometimes, however, it becomes clear to me that the best thing to do is to step aside. One of my patients, a young woman, was admitted to the ward with bizarre religious preoccupations. She was preparing, through diet and prayer, for an impending Armageddon. She heard voices that she understood as friendly spirits. She had pledged herself to a communal religious home where she said she felt safe. The patient's psychiatric history included treatment with a dozen antipsychotic medicines that had failed to blunt other hallucinations and delusions.

My initial instinct was to do something, to defend reality. But ultimately, I supported her discharge from the ward.

The fact was that whatever structure my patient's religious beliefs were providing was helping her, hallucinations and all, better than hospitals or medicines ever had.

Part of becoming a psychiatrist has been learning to use the techniques and tools at my disposal. Partnership with the law is an important one. Knowing how to use the courts is an invaluable skill in fighting mental illness.

An equal challenge, however, has been learning when to sit back, to listen to the wonderful, if sometimes painful, diversity of human experience, and to let well enough alone.

20

The Mask of Mania

A lifetime of happiness! No man alive could bear it; it would be hell on earth.

George Bernard Shaw   *Man and Superman*

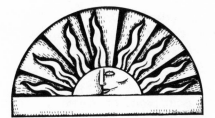

I hear I've got this new patient, and I'm looking around the hall for her. "She looks like an agency nurse," the ward secretary tells me. "She doesn't look like a patient."

Doesn't look like a patient. I readjust. Most of my patients are homeless and have stopped pretending they can take care of themselves. They're disheveled, and their eyes look tired from too much staring. Dark circles. Their teeth have gone bad. Their hair is cut unevenly so that it becomes funny- or tragic-looking, depending on whether the scalp is showing and whether there's any dried blood. I look for someone new who's put together pretty well. Like the staff. Like me.

I find her sitting in the community room at the end of the hall. She looks maybe fifty, perfectly attired in a gray wool skirt and white, ironed blouse, her hair silver and deliberately layered. She's reading a magazine through half-glasses. Normal picture, except for her boots. They're leather-and-rubber duck boots, the kind they sell at L. L. Bean, but they're missing the laces, and she's wearing them without socks.

"Mrs. Weissman?" I ask. I smile intentionally to appear kind.

Her head shoots up like a cork out of a bottle. "That's Miss Weissman. So you're my doctor," she laughs. "Yes you are. I knew it. I knew it." Her finger points at me staccato fashion every third word. "And another thing. Another thing. Don't you tell me what's going on with immigration. No, sir. I came here of my own free will. Now about the trial." She's looking over her shoulder as if someone's there, but no one is. Then she stands up and cocks her hip. "That little cutie at the nurse's station think she's putting one over. Well, I'll have you know . . . And I can tell you another thing. My sandals are at the Y. I paid twenty bucks for those things." She laughs. I notice her eyes are bright blue. Beautiful eyes. "Well, it's really a pleasure to meet you. What would Ayn Rand say about all this? I worked here once. Boston. Came back for the museum. Have you seen that museum? And what about Nathaniel Hawthorne?" Her hands are moving wildly in front of her. I take a step back. "Well, let me tell you." She reaches and pokes me with a finger, pauses nearly a second. "Now, where was I?"

Manic, I tell myself, proud of my quick assessment. Too much energy, too much speech, too many ideas. People with mania sleep too little, feel less hunger, and often have irrational and inflated views of their roles in the world. The flipside of depression. I'm already figuring how much lithium to start in someone her age. "The museum."

"Right. Was I? Well, anyhow. Now how am I supposed to get back to Rhode Island?" She waits for my answer, but her foot is tapping.

"I'll work on it," I say.

She smiles at me. "You'll work on it this year or next? I don't have forever, you know. There's special work to be done."

"This year," I smile back. We're having a little joke.

The admission note in her chart from the night doctor says she's come here on a bus from Rhode Island to see the Museum of Science, and she can't get back. So I spend three hours calling around and find out she's been a regular at the Rhode Island State Hospital since the late 1960s. Twenty-odd years in and out, always refusing to take medicine. Said to be highly intelligent. Finished school. Her family stopped being her family years ago, and she lives in shelters when they'll take her. Sometimes she hits people and gets thrown out—"barred," they call it. A doctor who took care of her once for four days tells me that she's "pleasantly crazy."

Well, she does seem pleasant. I mean, she's smiling, and you have to overstay your welcome pretty long before her eyes get all squinty, those glasses come off, and she starts in with the barbs. "Didn't I tell you I'm reading? You think you can just come in here. Well, I—And what about my sandals? You think I don't know how many times they've tried to lynch me? Just get out. Get out! And why don't you get a hairpiece while you're at it? And tell your parents I'll be sending them a bill for educating sonny boy."

She's all over the ward. Found a pink headband somewhere, and her hair is up off her forehead 1920s style. Everywhere I go, I see her. Walking fast. Laughing. Waving. Winking. We're starting to like having her around.

"She's a riot," one of the nurses nudges me.

"Fun," another adds.

Before long, we're all caught up in it. Mania is seductive stuff. All that energy is fun to watch. You can even start thinking the world might be a better place if there were more Miss Weissman's in it. I'm joking and winking back, and when she refuses to take her medicine, I figure I'm not going to force her. Nobody has for 20 years. "After all," I tell my supervisor, "Who are we to decide that someone has to take medicine if she's happy the way she is?"

I try asking her again, though. "Now, look," she says. She pokes me a couple times with her finger, but she's all smiles. "When you take care of that baldness of yours, I'll take your goddamn lithium. OK? OK? I mean, at your age. Really. You've got the disease, sonny. I like the way I am. Now get out. Out. Out."

I stop by later and invite her to attend group, and she shows. One of the patients is from Vietnam and misses his family back there. "I make friend. Mitsu. She my family now," Chan says. He's depressed and hears voices that tell him to hurt himself. He can't eat or sleep. "But I miss my real family."

"This is wonderful," Miss Weissman chimes in. She's looking from person to person and glancing occasionally skyward in thanks for the excitement. Her fists are clenched. "A real melting pot. Now I don't want to stay too long," she laughs, "but, really, it's all so interesting. What would Steinbeck have to . . . And you seem to be of Mexican descent. Am I right? I knew it. I knew it. Now don't let me go on too long. And you, I bet, from Africa. Mmm, hmm, mmm, hmm. If you think for one moment with these waves of immigration. Well, this is our future." Her arms stretch to indicate the group of patients.

"I don't have a-n-y family," another patient, Ed Bucco, smiles. He is big and slow-thinking, and when he laughs, his eyes get too wide and scare people. He feels hands touching his body when there are none there. "The only family I have is at West Home, and now I can't go back there 'cause I hit someone."

"My mother make me leave," Antonio Garcia nods.

"Why?" I ask. I know, but this group doesn't.

He looks down. "Drink."

I nod. "It must be very painful to be in the hospital without families to go home to," I say.

"Well, there you. You've hit the nail," Miss Weissman laughs. "What a melting pot." She straightens herself in her chair. "From all over. What would Kennedy say? Now you and you and you," she points. She's talking faster and faster. The thoughts are coming quicker than she can get them out. She's all smiles. "Now for me, I . . . And those sandals . . . Vietnam, you say . . . I'm telling you, the strong will inherit the earth. I'm . . . " Then, suddenly, the smile twitches, fades, and her face is all despair. She's crying. Quietly crying and embarrassed for it. "I'm sorry," she says, and straightens up again. "I'm sorry." Another tear builds and runs down her cheek.

The contrast between the excitement and tears jolts me. Surprises me. But it shouldn't. There's often a dark shadow in the gleam of mania—a terrible hurt, a festering self-esteem that needs the callus of euphoria to contain it, to stop it from eating everything away. I'd been caught up in the whirlwind of her illness, romanced into believing that the spectrum of what society calls normal might be simply too narrow. Too restrictive. Wonderful, these manic patients. I had let Miss Weissman's illness make me feel good, when her experience was anything but joyous.

21

Danger

Despite our best efforts to deny it, we all swim in that same chaotic sea of potentially violent emotions. We are all alone with the devil.

Ronald Markman, M.D.   *Alone With the Devil*

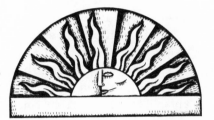

Protecting potential targets of my patients' aggression is one of the responsibilities as a senior resident in psychiatry. Although dangerousness is difficult to predict, there is a part of the routine psychiatric assessment that focuses on whether a person is thinking of harming—or even killing—someone.

It is a difficult question to ask, and I used to squint and say something like, "I hope you're not offended; I need to ask all my patients this: Have you had thoughts of harming anyone?"

The squint was a mix of embarrassment and fear. Tapping into someone's rage feels a lot like exploring his or her sexuality. Both are intensely private emotions, and even after nearly three years of residency, some remnant of the child in me still wonders what business it is of mine. Another part is afraid of the answer: that exploring such feelings, in fact, has become my stock in trade. I am responsible and, even more formidable, trusted to explore them.

In the face of possible risk to another person, I have a legal duty to either hospitalize a dangerous patient, alert the police or warn identifiable potential victims. This obligation is the result of a landmark 1974 malpractice decision by the California Supreme Court known as the *Tarasoff* case. Tatiana Tarasoff, a student at the University of California at Berkeley, was murdered by a graduate student who, disappointed that she was not responding to his romantic advances, told his psychiatrist that he fantasized about killing her. Although the psychiatrist notified university police, he did not contact city police, involuntarily hospitalize the patient or warn Tarasoff, whom the patient subsequently stabbed to death.

I have to check myself as the patient answers my questions about violence, because I always hope for a clear disavowal of violent intent. The promise of safety clarifies my allegiances, allowing me to focus my attention less on the outside world and more on the person seeking help. There is great comfort in the traditional confidentiality of the doctor-patient relationship, so much so that part of me would like to accept as sufficient an ambiguous response like, "I don't think I have it in me to ever really hurt him." Yet another more skeptical part of myself forces me to say: "I need to know if there is even a chance that you might."

Dangerousness is as much a feeling as a calculation. It takes its dimensions from a patient's past history, as well as current thoughts, appearance and behavior. One patient might talk openly of homicidal feelings toward a lover. Another may deplore violence but have his or her judgment clouded by psychosis. Still another, known to be seriously assaultive in the past, might come to the emergency room voluntarily—perhaps carrying a pocket knife—only to then refuse to answer questions.

There is a gravity in the moment when it becomes clear a patient cannot convince me that he or she is not a risk to others. It is as if an interpersonal hall of mirrors suddenly reveals a gaping new distance between us. I try closing it by reminding myself how frightening it must feel to be alone with so much rage. I can sometimes hear the patient's revelation as a plea to be held—literally and figuratively. Other times, on call without sleep, seeing the patient in the emergency room at 2 A.M., I think of the hours it can take to arrange for a bed on a locked ward. But I check myself, again.

Sometimes, I feel a duty to warn a potential victim even when the patient does not require further observation or hospitalization. A patient's promise that he or she won't hurt another person relies heavily on the patient's own appraisal of his or her self-control. Often, a patient is able to maintain self-control with the support and structure of a psychiatric ward. Some patients make threats when they are inebriated and then vehemently retract them following a night spent in the emergency room, after the alcohol has left their systems. "I said what? That's crazy," patients frequently tell me. "I was just drunk." But what about the next binge, I wonder?

Assessing dangerousness requires an appraisal of the patient's reliability. One person may confide violent fantasies that cross the line of confidentiality, while another may be utterly convincing in assuring me that thought will never turn to action.

I side with caution. I do not need to be convinced beyond a reasonable doubt of a patient's dangerousness. The doubt itself is reason enough for me to protect the community. I am not quick to risk my own safety, but I am slower still to risk the safety of others. The imprecision of this science engenders a healthy respect for the unpredictable.

I recall sitting in the center of a Boston emergency room last year, in a glass booth, doing paperwork. My patient had finally slept off his binge and assured me that his threat to kill his mother was just so much vodka. He loved her, he said, and would never hurt her.

I looked through the observation window at him, turned around and picked up the phone. I dialed, and that same embarrassment returned, the feeling that I was taking myself too seriously, playing emergency room psychiatrist. I wondered if I might be setting in motion an irrational chain of fear. Was murder really a possibility?

"I've been working with your son in the emergency room," I told the man's mother.

"He's been drinking again," she sighed. "Is he all right?"

"He's better now." I closed my eyes. "Actually, one reason I'm calling is to get your thoughts. When your son was intoxicated, he spoke of wanting to harm you," I said, squinting. "He even mentioned killing you. Has he ever hurt you physically?"

"Never. He'd never lay a hand on me. He talks nonsense sometimes. Send him home."

I continued: "He does seem calm now. He denies wanting to hurt you. But I wonder if you know how to get a restraining order, should you need one." I could feel that my face was flushed.

Since that night, I have had other, more personal, encounters with dangerousness. I have been assaulted by a state hospital patient who ended his flurry of punches with a simple, "No hard feelings"—and meant it. I have been threatened by an outpatient brandishing a knife. I have sat with people convicted of rape and murder who were perfectly pleasant to me. I have been shocked at hearing that patients whose names and faces I recognize from our wards or emergency rooms have gone on, in fact, to kill themselves or others.

And I have lost the embarrassment I used to feel when I found myself confronting what Freud called "the half-tamed demons that inhabit the human breast."

Now, I anticipate them. I don't think myself overly dramatic when I try to convey what seem even distant risks to the uninitiated. I know that the fear I sometimes inspire in potential victims is real and justified. I find myself repeating the warning, documenting it, checking to make sure that my new familiarity with danger does not make me jaded, immune to recognizing its subtleties or to communicating them.

22

Murder With
No Apparent Motive

In most forms of insanity lie elements of self-loathing that
can lead directly to self-punishment, self-destruction and,
sometimes, to destruction of others.

John F. Kappler, M.D.
"The Sounds of Terror and Laughter"
Los Angeles Times, 1978

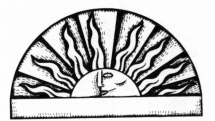

*I*t should come as no surprise that Dr. John Kappler finally took someone's life.

For over a decade, Kappler, an anesthesiologist, said voices instructed him to hurt other people. In 1975, he drove his car into another automobile on a California freeway. When the other driver got out of the car, Kappler took it and was involved in another accident. In 1980, the voices told him to administer the wrong drug during surgery to a patient who suffered a cardiac arrest. The patient recovered and no charges were filed. In 1985, he was charged with attempted murder for allegedly turning off the life support system to another patient; charges were dropped due to insufficient evidence, and Kappler retired from his practice shortly thereafter.

Last spring, Kappler was visiting Massachusetts from his home in California. On the afternoon of April 14, he later told police, the voices told him to drive his car onto a jogging path in Cambridge, killing my close friend and colleague Paul Mendelsohn. Kappler then accelerated and struck a 32-year-old single mother who was returning home from shopping. She survived with a broken pelvis and leg, as well as serious injuries to her face, head and neck. Kappler had apparently never met either victim and he ran from the scene.

At his murder trial, his lawyer introduced evidence that Kappler had been diagnosed, at various times since the 1960s, as suffering from schizophrenia, manic-depressive illness or atypical psychosis.

What Kappler took away is incalculable. Paul Mendelsohn would have been a chief resident in psychiatry at New England Medical Center in Boston this year. His gentle manner and tireless ear had helped him mature into someone colleagues already called a "doctor's doctor."

We had worked alongside one another through the grueling pressure of our internship year, becoming the kind of friends who hold pieces of each other within. Not long before he died, we had dinner. Paul was looking forward to returning home to California with his wife for the final six months of his training. We marveled at how quickly time was passing and agreed to spend more of it together.

But late on the night of April 14, an anesthesiology resident from Massachusetts General Hospital called me at home. The two of us had graduated from medical school together.

"We have a doctor in the intensive care unit, unconscious, who was jogging and got hit by a car," he said. "He was wearing a beeper from your psychiatry department. Who would have been carrying that today?"

"I don't know. What does he look like?" I asked.

"Well, that's just it. Between the accident and the work we did, there's too much swelling. Someone said he might be from California."

"My friend Paul Mendelsohn is from California," I replied. Even having spoken it, the link seemed unreal. Despite all the young people I have watched die painfully on medical wards, I irrationally reassured myself that Paul's death was unlikely because he was too good to die.

"We've heard it might be him," he started. "Listen, why don't I meet you in the hospital lobby? There are some other residents from your program here."

I hesitated. "Look, anyone from the program would know if it was Paul. He's tall with red hair," I argued.

"Keith, I don't think your friend's going to make it."

Paul was not technically dead when I arrived at the ICU. I could not recognize him. The leap—from a strong and healthy man of 32 to the disfigurement I saw before me—was incomprehensible. His life and his death seemed disconnected. Against nearly irrefutable evidence to the contrary, I fantasized a case of mistaken identity. My strongest image of that night is of walking his widow to his bedside and watching her draw back the bedsheet and identify him by the contour of his chest. I hadn't thought a woman could know a man by his chest.

The beeper became an instant symbol of death to me because it had helped the doctors identify Paul. I actually balked at accepting one from a colleague the next time I was on duty overnight.

I stayed at the ICU until early morning, not wanting to leave, as if my lingering could stop time. Kappler, meanwhile, had fled the scene of the accident on foot. He traveled to New York City and checked into a psychiatric hospital. He was returned to Massachusetts several days later to face trial for second-degree murder, assault and battery with a deadly weapon, driving to endanger and two counts of leaving the scene of an accident.

He pled not guilty. The voices, Kappler said, had plagued him again, this time insisting he drive up over the curb and onto the footpath to run down his victims.

I believe I wanted Kappler to be insane. At least that would allow me some understanding of the forces resulting in Paul's death. I would feel justified in allowing compassion for a sick person to mingle with my uncomfortable rage at his actions. I could let intellect buffer emotion.

At the same time, my mind took the liberty of painting Kappler as enormous and powerful, with danger in his eyes. It satisfied some illogical equilibrium in me that my friend's killer should be physically imposing enough to claim his life.

But when I attended his murder trial in Cambridge last December, I was disappointed to discover that the real Kappler was small and thin. His eyes were empty, and he seemed weak.

His trial lasted more than two weeks. After deliberating less than three hours, the jury found him guilty of all charges and sentenced him to life imprisonment. The verdict didn't hinge on the issue of whether Kappler was mentally ill. But it did turn on the question of whether he was legally insane at the moment that he drove his car onto the jogging path. Jurors decided he wasn't, possibly persuaded by the prosecution's argument that he had resisted previous commands by the voices, such as one that ordered him to commit suicide.

The verdict, predicated on Kappler's ability to choose right from wrong, leaves my intellect in uncharted territory. If I cannot explain his behavior as insanity, I am forced to contemplate what would lead someone to kill a person he has never met.

Everyone who has shared this tragedy with me has struggled with the same question. They still wonder what relationship John Kappler and Paul Mendelsohn might have had before the murder.

The desire for a connection is a plea for order in this fatal chaos, a bit of firm ground from which to view Kappler's motivation. If he wasn't crazy, I suppose we feel he should have been angry.

If John Kappler was neither, I am forced to confront the possibility of human evil, the idea that people might do terrible things to one another because they want to. Incarceration is one way our society tries to correct or contain that impulse. But like Gandhi, who conceived of all crime as illness, some would say that the only true cure is for the victims to love the perpetrators, to meet their evil with open arms and thereby render it impotent.

No one can say for sure what force took Paul Mendelsohn from this world. Nothing will bring him back. But if anyone was on his way to being able to absorb evil and survive with his soul intact, it was Paul.

23

Mental State

Our townsfolk were not more to blame than others; they forgot to be modest, that was all, and thought that everything still was possible for them. . . . They fancied themselves free, and no man will ever be free so long as there are pestilences.

Albert Camus *The Plague*

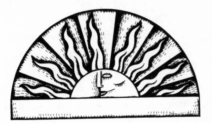

Morning rounds at Shattuck, the state mental hospital in Boston where I trained, would sometimes begin with an announcement of how many patients we had to discharge that day. The number of admissions had pushed the ward population too high to maintain reasonable and safe care. It was up to each of three treatment teams to select the healthiest patients to leave.

The problems of overcrowding and understaffing were real. Very sick patients bunked up to five in a room; some slept in the conference room. Many of us had been assaulted by patients in the past, and we could feel the ward get too "hot" when the number of patients got too high.

By discharging the "healthiest" patients, no one pretended that they were healthy. What we frequently meant was that the patients were believably disavowing any desire to kill themselves or others. Routinely, we discharged patients who, if they had money or insurance, would have stayed much longer in private hospitals.

These included those with continuing symptoms of severe depression, who were not actively suicidal; patients who were psychotic—out of touch with reality—but were not compelled by voices or hallucinations to commit violent acts; patients with limited understanding of their medications and those with nowhere to go but a shelter.

The selection of who would stay and who would go was partly subjective. Certain patients, by virtue of long-standing attachments to the ward staff or particularly evocative histories, were spared quick discharge. First episodes of mental illness, a recurrence of symptoms after a period of improvement or a background of education or professional achievement might lead to a longer stay. Believing that our care made a difference in these patients' lives, we made conscious decisions to "invest" in them.

One such patient was a battered wife in her forties. She had shown great strength in leaving her husband and overcoming her addiction to cocaine. In the wake of those triumphs, however, she experienced her first psychotic episode, believing that normal parts of her body were terribly deformed. She was not at immediate risk of suicide or a danger to others. Yet she remained on the ward for months, until her symptoms had resolved and a proper place for her to live had been found.

Any one of us—doctor, nurse, social worker—could object to a proposed discharge. Often the debate was passionate because the staff was made up of professionals who had made careers of helping people, not withholding care.

Even so, it seemed risky to argue for a longer stay. That might signal timidity or intransigence and would slow the wheels of the state mental health bureaucracy. By accident or design, we got the message: Good clinicians discharge quickly.

In this regard, I was better than most in keeping my caseload low. I constantly tried to distance the guilt I felt by telling myself that I was too overwhelmed with work even to attempt to fix the system.

That rationalization was an extension of the helplessness I began learning during my internship year. There had been enough nagging injustices, such as sleepless 30-hour shifts, that fighting them seemed futile. At some point, I decided it was triumph enough to just get through it.

Often, after expending much energy trying to persuade a reluctant patient to consent to further treatment, I found myself telling that person that he or she would be discharged the following morning. Sometimes, I said that the staff had reassessed the patient's condition. When that was clearly not true, I would admit that the ward was simply too crowded. Many patients correctly interpreted that as abandonment.

In some cases, it took repeated rehospitalizations in a short period to convince the treatment team to keep a patient longer than a few days. The patient had proved, no doubt painfully, that he or she couldn't make it. The investment seemed worthwhile if symptoms had worsened or if the alternative was the chaos—and paperwork—of frequent discharges and readmissions.

One such patient was an Asian refugee suffering from recurrent depression. Within one month, he was admitted twice complaining of suicidal thoughts. Both times, he improved in a few days and was discharged on antidepressants. We knew the medication might take several weeks to help lift the other symptoms of his depression. We knew that he had stopped taking the medicine when he was discharged. But it wasn't until his third admission in as many months that we committed ourselves to keeping him in the hospital long enough to monitor his mood and more fully address his lack of resources.

Not all my feelings were of helplessness. Part of my guilt arose from the fact that, although I was conscious of the unfairness of curbing admissions and facilitating discharges, I wanted fewer patients because I was overwhelmed and overworked. If I reduced the number of patients, I thought, I might be able to spend enough time with those remaining.

The rules of the game sparked turf wars between beleaguered hospitals. There was an art to finding holes in a transfer request from another ward or emergency room. The address might be phony. The patient might actually have some form of insurance which would require the transferring facility to document that no insured bed in the state was available.

Perhaps there was a distant military history, making the patient eligible for care in the Veterans Administration system. No detail was to be taken for granted. The same interrogation awaited us when we presented cases to other facilities. We had all been fooled once or twice into accepting patients who weren't "ours."

This mind-set probably caused fine cracks in my developing professional identity. It's hard to imagine that actively refining an ability to keep patients at bay would not seep into the doctor-patient relationship. As much as I was touched by many patients in the emergency room and on the ward, there was a conflicting benefit to sending them elsewhere. This paradox, not limited to state hospital patients, may have career-long effects on doctors and their patients.

The clinical setting may also have influenced me. The physical plant of Shattuck was frankly depressing. It seemed a clear statement that there were limits on the comfort to be afforded people who couldn't pay their way.

The clearest danger in all of this is that the patients who require the most care—those with major mental illness and few resources or advantages—often end up getting the least. This is no accident. Society keeps its distance from the overwhelming sadness of mental illness and our vulnerability to it.

Some people do this by conceiving of the homeless, for example, as vagrants or freeloaders or bums. The mean-spirited do it by poking fun at "crazies" or "nuts." As a group, we may do it by restricting health care resources. We close ranks in a kind of pathetic denial that we are all a certain number of crises away from needing that which we withhold from others.

24

Moral Insanity: Character and Mental Illness

Maybe we all have in us a secret pond where evil and ugly things germinate and grow strong. But this culture is fenced, and the swimming brood climbs up only to fall back. Might it not be that in the dark pools of some men the evil grows strong enough to wriggle over the fence and swim free? Would not such a man be our monster, and are we not related to him in our hidden water? It would be absurd if we did not understand both angels and devils, since we invented them.

John Steinbeck *East of Eden*

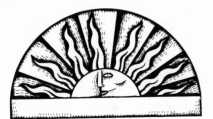

The security guard was visibly upset when I told him that the patient in the lobby, who had been discharged from the ward minutes before, would have to be escorted out of the hospital.

"He's bleeding," the guard said. "That's why I called you down here. He scraped himself with this coke can." The guard held up the ripped aluminum, as if to bring me to my senses. "You're saying I should *throw him out?*"

My patient, a 26-year-old man who had been diagnosed with borderline personality disorder, had repeatedly made superficial cuts on his arms in order to force us to keep him in the hospital. "Borderline" patients often feel chronically empty or bored and have unstable and intense interpersonal relationships. They may experience the end of hospitalization as abandonment and desperately attempt to remain on the ward. If consistently allowed to do so, they might regress beyond any hope of independence.

"Throw him out" was exactly what I was saying, but hearing it made me feel guilty. I tried to appear confident, even though I was frightened by the plan the treatment team and I had agreed upon.

"I know it doesn't seem to make sense," I told the bewildered guard, "but he has been told before that cutting himself won't make us postpone his discharge. He needs to leave."

"Whatever you say," the guard said warily, donning a pair of latex gloves to protect himself from the patient's blood. "But I'll need your name to write up an incident report."

With the patient screaming that I'd pay for my decision, the guard escorted him off the grounds.

I used to be confused by the seeming inability of the public to empathize with the mentally ill. The stigma associated with psychiatric illness seemed irrationally based on the idea that patients were weak or depraved rather than victims of illness. It was obvious to me that accidents of biology, not character flaws, were to blame.

After three years of training, I now see that psychiatry itself is unsure about how much responsibility many of our patients should bear for the way they interact with others. We tend to see patients who suffer from major mental illnesses, like depression or schizophrenia, as hostages to disease. We readily ally with those struggling to understand painful past events.

But when a patient's behavior seems to stem from a disorder of personality—an enduring, abnormal pattern of self-perception and of the ways one relates to other people—the lines of battle become less focused.

There is obvious confusion in the field about how much responsibility a patient should bear for being abnormally dependent, overly self-punishing or pathologically self-loving. Should people be held accountable for traits rooted in childhood trauma?

In 1830, James Pritchard, an English physician, identified this kind of "moral insanity," describing it as "madness consisting of a morbid perversion of the natural feelings, affections, inclinations, temper, habits and moral disposition, and natural impulses, without any remarkable disorder or defect of the intellect . . . and particularly without any insane illusion or hallucination."

Today, 11 separate disorders of personality, including paranoid and narcissistic, are listed in the official diagnostic manual by which psychiatrists classify patients. Yet little more is known about what causes them. Nor do we understand how to effectively treat them.

Indeed, many psychiatrists doubt that the current categories represent real and distinct conditions. The American Psychiatric Association's 3,000-page volume *Treatments of Psychiatric Disorders* acknowledges: "In 25 years, this diagnostic system may be unrecognizable by today's standards."

Partly for this reason, those who are functioning poorly as a result of their character or temperament, not from some clear-cut and disabling mental illness like schizophrenia, are only halfheartedly welcomed under the umbrella of psychiatry. Suspected of being able but unwilling to exert some control over their destructive interactions with others, they often spark an uncomfortable mixture of compassion, frustration and anger.

Working with patients with character disorders requires recognizing these troubling feelings. There are moments when I feel myself being drawn into conflict with a patient and then realize that I am responding in a way that rewards maladaptive behavior. Once I identify the trap, I am in a much better position to respond objectively and empathically, rather than becoming ensnared in an interpersonal tug of war.

Sometimes, however, symptoms of the patient's disorder cannot be tolerated within the structure of psychiatry.

This is often true for those diagnosed as having antisocial personality disorder. The official diagnostic criteria for this condition include inability to sustain employment, failure to honor financial obligations, no regard for truth, and acts, such as theft or assault, that are grounds for arrest.

Patients with the disorder are more likely than others to have been "hyperactive," truant from school, physically cruel to others and to have engaged in fire setting as children. They commonly have grown up in poor, single-parent families. And they are at much greater risk than the general population to die violently.

A patient I worked with a year ago fit the diagnosis. He had grown up in poverty, without a father, and was earning his money by selling drugs. He seemed to lie consistently, without any remorse. He repeatedly violated ward rules, swindling other patients out of their money and provoking physical fights. After being warned several times to stop, he was discharged.

Understanding his behavior as the logical outcome of a problematic childhood, even as consistent with a recognized disorder of character, was not enough to bring him the presumed innocence that typically accompanies the status of patient. We had diagnosed a psychiatric condition but were unprepared or unwilling to continue treating it in a psychiatric environment.

It is not uncommon for personality-disordered patients, engaged in a ceaseless battle with the health care system, to be admitted and discharged hundreds of times during their lives.

Many become wards of the penal system. Jails are filled with personality-disordered inmates. Whether or not an inability to appreciate the suffering of others and a preoccupation with unlimited power—symptoms of narcissistic personality disorder—lurk in the background of a crime, the perpetrator is considered a criminal, not a patient. Without known organic abnormalities such as a seizure disorder at the root of disordered character, we balk at conceiving of a person's harmful actions as an inescapable chapter in his or her life story.

It is not clear that psychiatry is the preferred custodian. First, we have no proven treatment to offer. Second, labeling people as sick, rather than as criminal, could make psychiatry an unwitting enforcer of social mores, a perversion of what medicine is supposed to be. Perhaps we would miss entirely the possibility that personality disorders reflect a defective social structure, rather than defective individuals.

This is not a new dilemma. It is at the core of Dostoevsky's Raskolnikov and Camus' Mersault, fictional murderers who, lacking the ability to appreciate the suffering of others, seem morbidly compelled to do evil.

As psychiatry continues to bring science to the subject of character, we will be forced to reconcile the philosophical and spiritual dimensions, as well. In doing so, we may rediscover that they are, no less than pharmacology, our proper domain.

25

Safe Passage: Psychotherapy and the Status Quo

"But I don't want comfort. I want God, I want poetry, I want real danger, I want freedom, I want goodness. I want sin."

"In fact," said Mustapha Mond, "you're claiming the right to be unhappy."

"All right then," said the Savage defiantly, "I'm claiming the right to be unhappy."

"Not to mention the right to grow old and ugly and impotent . . . the right to be lousy . . . the right to be tortured by unspeakable pains of every kind." There was a long silence.

"I claim them all," said the Savage at last.

Aldous Huxley *Brave New World*

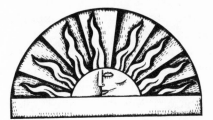

*E*arly in therapy, a young woman I treated for depression described her ideal relationship with a man.

"If I had my way," she said, "I wouldn't do a thing, except clean the house and talk on the phone. He would make all the decisions. He would pick where we go, what we do, who we see."

Because I have been taught that independence is both psychologically healthy and personally rewarding, I immediately doubted that my patient could truly be content with the lifestyle she had described. "Have you ever had a relationship like that?" I asked skeptically.

"Until he broke it off," she said. "But I'd go back in a second."

My mind went through the mental data base of diagnoses I have memorized from the official diagnostic manual published by the American Psychiatric Association. I began to think that she was suffering from *dependent personality disorder*, a condition marked by low self-esteem and submissive behavior. I resolved that whatever the diagnosis, the success of therapy would be measured partly by an increase in her self-reliance.

After her depression had lifted, I helped her to find the roots of her unusually dependent feelings in the lack of safety she experienced as a child of violent, unpredictable parents. She was interested in the connection, but she also made it clear that it was not her goal to become independent.

"If I have to, I guess I'll work," she said. "But I'd rather do nothing. That's what I like." She paused and smiled. "Does that make me crazy?"

The answer to that question might depend more on prevailing public opinion than on science. Three years into psychiatric training, I have yet to help a patient become personally comfortable with a stated desire that runs dramatically counter to contemporary social values.

The value our society places on independence, achievement, law-fulness and honesty flows so freely into therapy that I worry about becoming an unwitting proponent—and subtle enforcer—of main-stream thought and behavior.

I am aware that I embody and ascribe to those values. As someone drawn to the medical profession, with its rigid hierarchy and emphasis on academic honesty, I began my training already comfortable with conventional expectations. My ability to complete over a decade of regimented study confirmed my prowess at working independently, meeting deadlines and deferring gratification. Merely by my example, I could be relied upon to give voice to some of what our society cherishes.

I have been supported in this by the inherent structure of psychiatric care. Helping patients look for hidden meaning—such as displaced anger—in lateness to appointments, for example, reinforces the idea that punctuality reflects emotional health, when in fact it might indicate compulsiveness or even obsequiousness.

Presenting the exchange of money as an essential component of the therapeutic relationship tends to legitimize only those things that can be bought.

On the psychiatric inpatient wards where I trained, all patients were made to progress through a series of privileges, reinforcing the notion that satisfying authority figures is a prerequisite for freedom.

This role as social gatekeeper is not new to psychiatry. By the early 1900s, leaders in the field were anxious to exert influence beyond the walls of mental hospitals. They hoped that psychotherapy could be an agent for the betterment of society, an instrument of social change that would ameliorate problems such as alcoholism, prostitution and delin-quency.

My discomfort comes from the fact that these subjective goals are largely unstated today. Yet they are clearly incorporated in the diagnos-tic categories by which we classify patients. In rushing to use the language of medicine—forgetting we carry with us a heritage steeped in morality—we run the risk of defining socially accepted conduct as health and unfashionable or unconventional lifestyles as disease.

The fact is that psychiatry does not change simply through scientific discovery. Our perspective as clinicians changes with the times. Not so many decades ago, when attitudes toward women were different, certain behaviors, such as assertiveness, which would now be considered normal, were regarded as neurotic. In the 1950s, my patient's yearning for a completely dependent lifestyle would probably not have been thought pathological in the least.

More recently, homosexuality was listed as a mental illness by the American Psychiatric Association in the late 1970s; by the early 1980s that was no longer the case. Changing public attitudes fueled by various civil rights movements of the 1960s and 1970s, not new scientific discoveries, led to a major change in the way most psychiatrists regard and treat gay men and women. The current classification is *sexual disorder not otherwise specified*, in which reference to the word homosexual is avoided by defining the condition as "persistent and marked distress about one's sexual orientation."

The entire domain of personality disorders, conditions in which patients display enduring patterns of conduct that limit their functioning at work or in social situations, incorporates a Western work ethic. The American Psychiatric Association's diagnostic manual describes *passive-aggressive personality disorder*, for example, as follows:

> People with this disorder habitually resent and oppose demands to increase or maintain a given level of functioning. This occurs most clearly in work situations, but is also evident in social functioning. The resistance is expressed indirectly through such maneuvers as procrastination, dawdling, stubbornness, intentional inefficiency, and "forgetfulness." These people obstruct the efforts of others by failing to do their share of the work.

Diagnostic criteria for other personality disorders include truancy from school, theft, lying, drug use and lack of friends.

There is no question that such patients suffer because they are social outcasts. The danger is that contemporary psychiatry, with its increasing emphasis on biology, tends to think differently about disease and, by extension, about them. The view that abnormal brain structure and chemistry lie at the root of many disorders means that psychiatrists can easily lend a very powerful sense of what is normal to subjective social and behavioral standards.

There are lessons to be culled from some of the symptoms and behavior of disturbed patients.

A man I treated for mania, a mental illness marked by grandiose behavior, increased energy and social indiscretions, was in the habit of giving his money away to anyone who asked.

"You've got to stop giving out money on the street," I told him, referring to his propensity to walk up to complete strangers and hand them a five-dollar bill.

"Stop? Why?" he asked incredulously. "I only give away what I don't need."

I smiled at the thought that my patient's values, even though they were a symptom of his illness, might be lauded in a more just world.

"That's a noble thought," I said. "But people won't know what to make of it. Someone who sees you giving away some of your money might hurt you to get the rest of it."

In patients like the dependent young woman may also be a hope for a kind of intimacy most of us fear and a lesson in the limits of rugged individualism.

Maybe some people fail to meet social demands because the demands themselves are flawed.

I don't believe in the least that psychiatry intends to stifle social change, limit diversity or punish unconventional behavior. But as we build a foundation in hard science, we should not forget that many of the planks from which we speak with such authority and apparent objectivity are still hewn from morality and ethics.